Biobanking of Human Biospecimens

Pierre Hainaut • Jim Vaught
Kurt Zatloukal • Markus Pasterk
Editors

Biobanking of Human Biospecimens

Lessons from 25 Years of Biobanking Experience

Second Edition

Springer

Editors
Pierre Hainaut
Institute for Advanced Biosciences
La Tronche, France

Kurt Zatloukal
Diagnostic and Research Center
for Molecular BioMedicine
Medical University of Graz
Graz, Steiermark, Austria

Jim Vaught
International Prevention Research Institute
Editor-in-Chief, Biopreservation
and Biobanking
Kensington, MD, USA

Markus Pasterk
Science and Research
Austrian Federal Ministry of Education and
University of Milano-Bicocca, Milan, Italy
Vienna, Austria

ISBN 978-3-030-55900-7 ISBN 978-3-030-55901-4 (eBook)
https://doi.org/10.1007/978-3-030-55901-4

This Springer imprint is published by the registered company Springer Nature Switzerland AG
The registered company address is: Gewerbestrasse 11, 6330 Cham, Switzerland

Preface

Over the past 25 years, biobanks of human specimens have become a cornerstone for research on human health and have empowered the "omics" revolution that characterizes biomedical science in the twenty-first century. Today, biobanking of human specimens is a critical component of the interface between clinical practice and translational research, supporting the discovery and validation of new biomarkers of disease etiology, risk, early detection, diagnosis, prognosis, prediction, and relapse. Today, biobanking is a foundation for personalized medicine, enabling clinical investigations on genetic, transcriptomic, proteomic, metabolomic, and immunological biomarkers useful to inform caregivers for therapeutic decisions. Data generated from biobanks represent a rapidly growing and highly valuable resource, participating in the emergence of Big Data Medicine. With the development of large computing capabilities and artificial intelligence, data associated with biobanked specimens constitute a resource of exceptional interest for the discovery and validation of new biomarkers and therapeutically actionable targets. Interconnecting, interoperating, and sharing this data is a major issue for national health systems, raising enormous stakes as well as major societal, ethical, legal, and cybersecurity challenges in terms of compliance with the protection of personal sensitive information.

So far, there has been a lack of major textbooks on biobanking. Documentation for biobanking is widely available through numerous publications, regulatory documents published by international or governmental agencies, and sets of recommendations essentially accessible through the Internet. However, it is difficult to access a single, top-of-the-shelf reference that provides at a glance a large coverage of all aspects of human biobanking. Fulfilling this need is the main origin of the concept for this publication project. This book is the second part of an initiative launched in 2012 to produce a published corpus of knowledge encompassing all aspects of human biobanking as a central practice for research and medicine. The overarching aim is to provide a "one-stop shop" for practical state-of-the-art information on what constitutes the field of human biobanking, from conception of a biobank,standard operating procedures, ethical and societal aspects, governance, networking, interoperability, and economic sustainability.

The first volume, published in 2017, is entitled: *Human Biobanking: Principles and Practice*. It focuses on key principles for establishing a biobank, safety and economic issues, types of biobanks, networking and worldwide deployment of biobanks in different countries and socio-economic contexts. This new book constitutes Volume 2 of the same initiative and is entitled *Biobanking of Human Biospecimen: Lessons from 25 Years of Biobanking Experience*. The aim of this second volume is to compile practical lessons and best practice recommendations drawn from 25 years of experience in biobanking by international experts. Hence, the two volumes complement each other while having their specificities in terms of what they actually cover. As a result, the two books are "twins" but can also be used independently of each other.

The general theme of this second volume is biobanking as cornerstone for biomarker discovery, as underlined in the opening chapter by Jim Vaught. Next, the volume addresses practical issues in biobank design and engineering (Chap. 2, Pasquale de Blasio and Mario Conconi) and in developing biocomputing information management systems for biobanks (Chap. 3, Cheryl Michels). Next, two chapters are dedicated to specimen quality and tissue preservation issues (Chap. 4, Peter Riegman and Chap. 5, Giorgo Stanta and Serena Bonin, addressing the use of pathology archives). In Chap. 6, Jim Vaught discusses the development of biospecimen research as a specific R&D topic and reflects on 20 years of experience in formulating best practices. Chaps. 7 and 8 provide complementary views and opinions on the complexity of ethical, legal, and societal issues (ELSI) surrounding biobanks. In Chap. 7, Kirsi Vähäkangas and colleagues propose an extensive review and opinion piece on practical ethical questions faced by scientists involved in collecting, storing, and using biospecimens. Chapter 8 (Lawrence and colleagues) describes a unique initiative for developing an academic cursus for training biobank managers at Master level, supporting the emergence of a specific professional qualification. Chapters 9 and 10 draw lessons from initiatives for developing biobank networks at national and international level. In Chap. 9, Manuel Morente and colleagues reflect on their building of national network in Spain, whereas in Chap. 10, Peter Abuja and Kurt Zatloukal explain the structure and development of the European biobanking infrastructure (BBMRI-ERIC). As a final note, a chapter written by the editors outlines a prospective vision of the future of biobanking and of the challenges ahead.

Together, these 11 chapters compile a vast amount of practical information and recommendations for setting-up and managing a biobank and therefore constitute a unique source of expert advice for all actors and stakeholders in the biobanking field. The inclusive approach meets the needs of a vast readership, including scientists, doctors, and technical staffs who are directly involved in biobanking operations, scientists in other disciplines that heavily rely on biobanking (such as genomics or proteomics), stakeholders and policy makers, and of course students for whom biobanking is becoming an important part of the training curriculum.

La Tronche, France
Kensington, MD, USA
Graz, Steiermark, Austria
Vienna, Austria

Pierre Hainaut
Jim Vaught
Kurt Zatloukal
Markus Pasterk

Contents

Chapter 1
Biobanking for Biomarker Discovery

Jim Vaught

Abstract The implementation of personalized or precision medicine involves developing therapeutic agents to fit a patient's molecular profile. Biomarkers are defined as "any characteristic that can be objectively measured and evaluated as an indicator of normal biological processes, pathogenic processes, or pharmacological response to a therapeutic intervention." Biomarkers typically undergo discovery and development phases. In biomarker discovery or development, the laboratory assays for the markers must be standardized in a way that results are comparable among a variety of laboratories. The importance of a standardized, well-controlled approach to biospecimen management and biobank operation to biomarker discovery is also well-established. A multitude of factors including preanalytical variables can affect biospecimen quality and as a result the analyses necessary to discover and validate biomarkers. Biospecimens of consistent quality are necessary as critical starting materials for biomarker discovery and the clinical assay development processes. Biobanks that serve as sources of biospecimens for biomarker studies should adhere to best practices such as those developed by international biobanking organizations. The importance of biobanking standards in biomarker discovery and development has also been recognized in several sets of recommendations and guidelines for authors, reviewers, and editors.

Keywords Biobanking · Biomarker · Biospecimen · Preanalytical variables · Precision medicine · Personalized medicine · Molecular diagnostics · Genomics

1.1 Biomarkers and Personalized Medicine

The era of personalized or precision medicine promises that therapy can be tailored to fit an individual patient's molecular profile [1]. Biomarkers have been defined as "any characteristic that can be objectively measured and evaluated as an indicator of normal biological processes, pathogenic processes, or pharmacological response to a therapeutic intervention" [1]. Biomarkers can be classified as: diagnostic, for early detection and disease classification; predictive, to predict a patient's likely response,

J. Vaught (✉)
International Prevention Research Institute, Kensington, MD, USA

P. Hainaut et al. (eds.), *Biobanking of Human Biospecimens*,
https://doi.org/10.1007/978-3-030-55901-4_1

either positive or adverse; metabolic, to define treatment dosage; and outcome, to forecast response, progression, and recurrence [2]. In this chapter, most of the examples of the involvement of biobanking and biospecimens in biomarker discovery are from the cancer research field. However, the discussion is relevant to all categories of diseases and their respective biomarkers.

For example, HER2/neu is part of a group of ErbB transmembrane receptor tyrosine kinases and is an example of a predictive biomarker [3]. HER2 overexpression is used to categorize breast cancer patients with aggressive disease with a poor prognosis and unlikely to respond to standard therapies. Such patients are candidates for treatment with Herceptin [3]. Issues related to laboratory analyses of HER2 and the effects of preanalytical variables in the collection and processing of tissues for the analyses will be discussed later in this chapter.

1.2 Discovery Versus Development of Biomarkers

Biomarkers typically undergo discovery and development phases [4]. In the discovery phase, cancer biomarker research is "oriented toward the identification of novel markers that may be important drivers or other indicators of malignant transformation and/or neoplastic progression" [4]. Clinical biomarker development is oriented to directing therapy or measuring a clinical outcome.

In biomarker discovery or development, the laboratory assays for the markers must be standardized in a way that results are comparable among a variety of laboratories. However, there are differences in this regard, depending on whether the biomarker assay results will be used for clinical decision-making or not. In the case of "integral" markers that are used for clinical decision-making, in the US a Clinical Laboratory Improvement Amendment (CLIA) certified laboratory must be used [4]. Becoming CLIA-certified means that laboratory assays are generally more reproducible and reliable when performed in multiple settings. However, in the case of biomarker discovery research that is performed in an academic laboratory, the process for developing and implementing assays is not well-regulated. As a result, the collection and processing of biospecimens (blood, tissue) necessary for the assays are often not controlled in a manner that will lead to reliable analyses [4]. An example of issues that can arise when biospecimens are randomly chosen from existing biobanks for a multi-institution study comes from NIH's The Cancer Genome Atlas [5], discussed next, in Sect. 1.3.

1.3 The Cancer Genome Atlas

As noted on its website [5] The Cancer Genome Atlas (TCGA): "began as a three-year pilot in 2006 with an investment of $50 million each from the U.S. National Cancer Institute (NCI) and National Human Genome Research Institute (NHGRI).

The TCGA pilot project confirmed that an atlas of changes could be created for specific cancer types. It also showed that a national network of research and technology teams working on distinct but related projects could pool the results of their efforts, create an economy of scale and develop an infrastructure for making the data publicly accessible. Importantly, it proved that making the data freely available would enable researchers anywhere around the world to make and validate important discoveries. The success of the pilot led the National Institutes of Health to commit major resources to TCGA to collect and characterize more than 20 additional tumor types." A number of publications have resulted from TCGA biomarker discovery efforts [6, 7].

However, the ultimate success of TCGA was preceded in the pilot phase by a period where a large proportion of the biospecimens did not qualify for inclusion in the study [2]. The project initially required that frozen tissue specimens meet stringent criteria, including 80% viable tumor nuclei and minimal necrotic areas, to meet the standards required by the analytic platforms at the time of the study initiation. Preliminary contacts and site visits to biobanks with large numbers of the pilot study target tumor samples (glioblastoma multiforme, serous ovarian and lung squamous cell tumors) indicated that more than enough samples were available from existing collections. However, the initial pathology and molecular quality control processes eliminated the majority of samples from further analysis.

The early failure to accrue sufficient samples for TCGA was the result of several factors. The samples in existing (retrospective) biobanks were not collected with the intention of using them for a project with requirements such as those for TCGA. But this is indicative of a larger issue, i.e., biospecimens are not generally collected, processed, and stored under consistent strict standards that will result in their suitability for broad use in genomic, proteomic, and other analytical applications [8]. The early biospecimen quality failures in TCGA resulted in a new approach where samples were collected prospectively under strict standard operating procedures. As a result, the quality control pass rate increased dramatically (Fig. 1.1).

One of the results of the initial low pass rate for TCGA samples was that funds were wasted collecting and performing quality control analyses on samples that failed. The average cost for collecting TCGA samples and data was about $2000 for each case (tumor sample, control tissue or blood, and clinical data). Since a significant amount of time was required for pathologists and biobank staff to retrieve and process samples and data even if the case submission ultimately failed quality control, the costs were justifiable. However, since every 500 samples that failed to enter TCGA's analysis pipeline cost about $1,000,000 to collect and process, the economic consequences were significant. As a result of the implementation of the prospective collection of samples, significant cost savings are projected. See Chap. 3 (Economics of Biobanking), 1st edition, for additional discussion of the financial impact of various biobank management approaches.

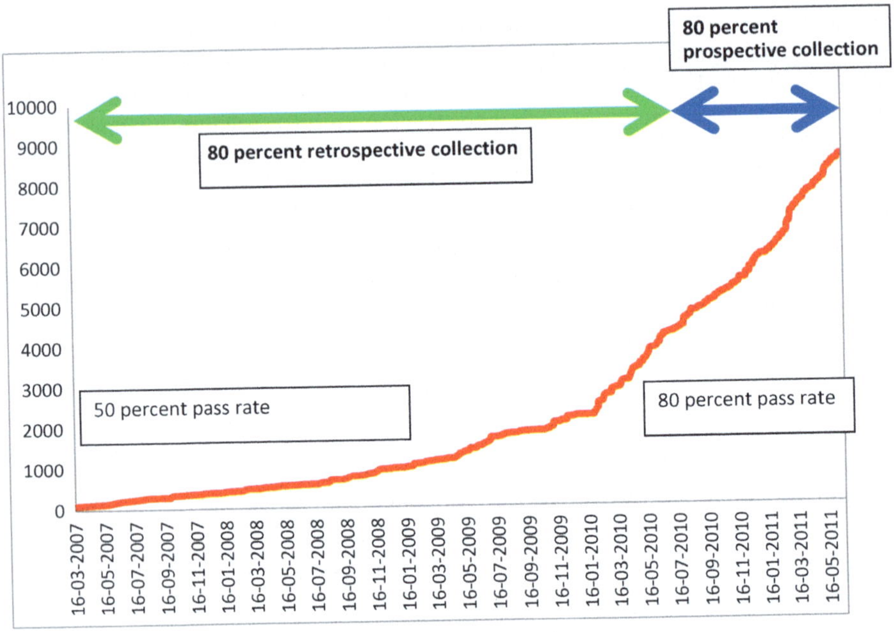

Fig. 1.1 The Cancer Genome Atlas. Quality control pass rate improves as *prospective collection* using best practices/SOPs is implemented. (*Courtesy of NCI TCGA Program Office*)

1.4 Sample Types for Biomarker Development

Biospecimens for biomarker discovery and development can encompass tissue samples including formalin-fixed paraffin-embedded, frozen tissue, and tissue microarrays; and liquid samples including blood and blood fractions (serum, plasma, whole blood) as well as urine. Each of these sample types will have special considerations that need to be taken into account when using them for biomarker studies [8]. And within the various sample types, derivative samples such as DNA, RNA, and protein also have specific processing and quality requirements that should be followed to optimize biomarker assay development.

It should be noted that tissue samples come in a variety of types including frozen, formalin-fixed, paraffin-embedded, and tissue microarrays. Each of these sample types must be evaluated for the variables specific to the analytical platforms to be used. Although tissue microarrays have been used for many years for biomarker studies, recent developments in automated microarray construction and digital pathology have led to "next-generation tissue microarray" technology, requiring new considerations for optimizing biomarker studies using such samples [9].

Although most biomarker development continues to be performed using the traditional methods and with tissue, blood, and urine as the specimens of choice, recent developments in, for example, circulating tumor cells and other single-cell analytical techniques [10] will increasingly lead to their use in metabolomics and biomarker development. As for other sample types, preanalytical variables that may affect biomarker assay discovery and development will need to be assessed as these samples are increasingly used.

1.5 Preanalytic Factors in Biomarker Discovery and Development

In recent years, the effects of preanalytic variables on the quality of biospecimens and their downstream analyses have gained a lot of attention [11, 12]. The US NCI Biorepositories and Biospecimen Research Branch [11], as well as the Biobanking and Biomolecular Research Infrastructure (BBMRI) and Standardisation and Improvement of generic pre-analytical tools and procedures for in-vitro diagnostics (SPIDIA) [13, 14] have been among the leaders in identifying biospecimen preanalytic variables as an important area of research. NCI has hosted several biospecimen research symposia [15] that address the major issues surrounding evidence-based approaches to biospecimen collection, processing, and storage. Organizations such as the International Society for Biological and Environmental Repositories (ISBER) and European, Middle Eastern and African Society for Biopreservation and Biobanking (ESBB) now include "biospecimen research" as a category in their conferences. ISBER has a biopecimen research working group that has published a number of papers [16].

In general, the preanalytical variables that may affect biospecimen quality and analysis are fairly straightforward. Some examples are time to fixation or freezing after collection (cold ischemic time); timing and duration of tissue fixation; stabilization method (freezing, fixation); storage temperature; number of thawing and refreezing cycles; and additives to blood-collection tubes (e.g., EDTA, heparin, citrate). Of course, not all of these variables will affect sample quality or analysis as the assessment of such studies has shown [17].

However, as noted by Hewitt et al. [8], the factors that have traditionally been used to evaluate tissue quality for histopathological applications are not necessarily applicable to molecular applications [8, 18]. Methods that may properly preserve tissues for clinical diagnostic purposes may compromise the biomolecules necessary for biomarker discovery and development. Hewitt et al. [8] outline a series of "first-order" and "second-order" biospecimen issues that need to be considered for biomarker discovery and development (Tables 1.1 and 1.2, [8]). Among these are the intended use of the biomarker assay; the type of biospecimen (tissue, fluid); stability of the samples under the storage conditions; replicability of the assay in various laboratories; the minimum samples size necessary; preanalytical variables to consider; and sources of assay interference.

As noted in the introduction, the analysis of HER2 and the resulting treatment of HER2-positive patients with Herceptin became an issue when it was determined that a significant number of false positives and false negatives were occurring, up to

Table 1.1 Examples of first-order biospecimen issues for new biomarkers (From Reference [8], reprinted with permission)

What is the intended use of the assay?
What is the clinical utility (how useful is the diagnostic for its intended clinical use)?
What additional information is required for an accurate test result?
What biomolecule or analyte is being analyzed?
What types of tissue/fluid will be used for analysis?
Does a clinical specification exist for this biospecimen?
Is this specification adequate for this test?
Have the specimens been serially tested to determine whether they are stable in storage?
Can the assay be replicated in another laboratory with the original specimens?
Can the assay be replicated in the original laboratory with submitted specimens?

Table 1.2 Examples of second-order biospecimen issues for new biomarkers (From Reference [8], reprinted with permission)

What is the minimum specimen size?
What quantities are involved (e.g., microliters of fluid, micrograms of tissue, number of cells)?
Are nonstandard specimen-handling procedures required?
Are frozen tissues, alternative fixatives, or nonroutine blood-collection tubes required?
Have common variables of biospecimen handling been tested as a source of assay variability?
What are some issues involving fluids (e.g., temperature, time, separation technologies)?
What are some issues involving tissues (e.g., fixative, fixation times, processing times, specimen storage)?
Have other analytes been shown to interfere with the assay?
Is a document available that specifies an adequate vs. inadequate biospecimen for this assay?

20% in some reviews of laboratory results. False positives resulted in undue stress for patients, as well as unnecessary expensive and potentially toxic treatments. False negatives could result in missing aggressive breast tumor diagnoses. A review of the HER2 analysis issues by the College of American Pathologists (CAP) and the American Society for Clinical Oncology (ASCO) found that among the root causes of the discrepant assays was the variability of tissue collection and fixation times and other biospecimen-related issues. In 2007 [19] ASCO and CAP jointly published an article that recommended that strict biospecimen collection and processing protocols be followed to prevent such large discrepancies and interlaboratory variation in HER2 analyses. The guidelines were recently updated [20]. A 2013 update suggests that the situation has improved during the 6 years following the initial 2007 ASCO/CAP guidelines publication [21].

1.6 Recommendations for Biobanking Standards for Biomarker Discovery and Development

A number of best practices documents have been produced in recent years to better standardize biospecimen management. Among the most widely adopted are those from ISBER, the US NCI, OECD, IARC, and others [22]. These best practices address the most critical issues relating to biospecimens and biobanks, including initial establishment and operation of a biobank; technical approaches to sample collection, processing, analysis, storage, shipment; data collection and processing for sample inventory and tracking purposes, as well as clinical annotation and sample analyses; ethical and regulatory issues such as informed consent, intellectual property, privacy, material transfer, return of research results; and business practices and economic factors related to biobank development and sustainability.

More specific to biobanks as they apply to biomarker research, as part of work of the American Association for Cancer Research-FDA-NCI Cancer Biomarkers Collaborative, Khleif et al. [2] produced a set of consensus recommendations that recognized biospecimens as critical resources for biomarker discovery and validation in cancer drug development. The categories (adapted from Khleif et al. [2]) of these recommendations are biospecimens; analytic performance; standardization and harmonization; bioinformatics; collaboration and data sharing; regulatory issues; Stakeholder education and communication; and science policy. The Biospecimens category recommends:

- Establish quality standards and promote routine quality assessment of biospecimens acquired for research.
- Develop a publicly available national oncology resource of biospecimen reference standards for biospecimen quality assessment.
- Promote an infrastructure and climate supportive of biospecimen research.

The other categories among these recommendations also have multiple references to biospecimen research and implementation of quality standards and availability of reference materials. Some of these recommendations have been partially implemented in various programs in the US, Europe, and elsewhere, but much remains to be done to achieve national and international adherence to such recommendations.

The importance of biobanking standards in biomarker discovery and development has also been recognized in several sets of recommendations and guidelines for authors, reviewers, and editors. For example, the Reporting Recommendations for Tumor Marker Prognostic Studies (REMARK [23]), includes among its materials and methods recommendations several direct and indirect references to reporting on biospecimen collection and analysis parameters. Similarly, Biospecimen Reporting for Improved Study Quality, published simultaneously in three journals in 2011 (BRISQ [24]), includes guidelines concerning biospecimen collection, stabilization, processing, and storage conditions that should be reported by authors in their manuscripts, and considered important for reviewers and journal editors to evaluate before publishing papers. BRISQ recommendations are organized into three tiers, tier 1 being the minimal set of sample collection and processing conditions that should be reported, and tiers 2 and 3 being information on conditions that are less likely to be routinely monitored and reported.

The reason that guidelines such as BRISQ and REMARK are necessary is that investigators tend not to provide sufficient details concerning the samples used in their analyses. This tendency is one of the reasons that the effects of preanalytical variables on biomarker research have not been more thoroughly clarified. See reference [25] for an assessment of reporting of biospecimen variables in several journals.

The US NCI Clinical Assay Development Program [26, 27] was established to enable independent academic and small-company investigators to develop clinically rigorous assays that can then enter clinical trials for clinical qualification and ultimately assessment of clinical utility. The CADP fulfills a need in the biomarker research community due to the issues outlined in this chapter that result from biospecimens being of inconsistent quality, resulting in issues with their use in molecular diagnostics analyses. As noted by Williams et al. [27] "it is often difficult to validate novel biomarker assays due to the lack of a gold standard assay." The NCI CADP addresses this issue by providing services that match investigators in need of validation of their assays with CLIA-certified laboratories. Such a service improves the reliability of assays that will be used for clinical diagnostic and prognostic purposes.

1.7 Conclusion

Biomarker discovery and development and their importance in personalized medicine are now well-established. The importance of a standardized, well-controlled approach to biospecimen management and biobank operation to biomarker discovery is also well-established. The issues discussed in this chapter show how a multitude of factors can affect biospecimen quality and as a result the analyses necessary to discover and validate biomarkers. A variety of excellent studies have been conducted that have helped to refine the nature of these factors and variables. Specific recommendations have resulted such as the ASCO-CAP guidelines for HER2 analysis. Broader guidelines such as REMARK and BRISQ show promise in terms of showing investigators, authors, reviewers, and editors the importance of biospecimens and biobanking approaches to biomarker research. In addition, CAP recently introduced its Biorepository Accreditation Program [28] that is in the process of assessing and providing formal accreditation to biobanks, according to a set of criteria based on ISBER, NCI, and other best practices as well as CAP-developed standards. Such accreditation programs will over time contribute to improvements in the standardization of specimen quality for biomarker discovery and development as well as other applications.

However, the number of preanalytical variables and other biospecimen factors that may influence biomarker discovery and development are numerous. Most of these factors have not been studied in detail. Since much of the research enterprise is now global in nature, what is needed is better international coordination and collaboration to establish and implement best practices for biospecimen management and biomarker assay development and validation. Progress is being made in these areas, and the reader is referred to organizations such as ISBER, ESBB, the US NCI Clinical Assay Development Program, and similar initiatives [28–30]. In addition, see the volume published by the International Agency for Research on Cancer, Unit 2, "Biomarkers: practical aspects" [31], where many of the issues discussed in this chapter are discussed with respect to biospecimen management and analysis for biomarker discovery and development.

References

1. Nass SJ, Moses HL (2007) Cancer biomarkers. The promises and challenges of improving detection and treatment. The National Academies Press, Washington, DC
2. Khleif SN, Doroshow JH, Hait WN (2010) AACR-FDA-NCI cancer biomarkers collaborative consensus report: advancing the use of biomarkers in cancer drug development. Clin Cancer Res 16:3299–3318
3. Taube SE, Clark GM, Dancey JE et al (2009) A perspective on challenges and issues in biomarker development and drug and biomarker codevelopment. J Natl Cancer Inst 101:1453–1463
4. Poste G, Carbone DP, Parkinson DR et al (2012) Leveling the playing field: bringing development of biomarkers and molecular diagnostics up to the standards for drug development. Clin Cancer Res 18:1515–1523
5. The Cancer Genome Atlas. US National Human Genome Research Institute: http://cancergenome.nih.gov/abouttcga/overview. Accessed 15 Feb 2021
6. The Cancer Genome Atlas Research Network (2008) Comprehensive genomic characterization defines human glioblastoma genes and core pathways. Nature 455(7216):1061–1068
7. The Cancer Genome Atlas Research Network (2011) Integrated genomic analyses of ovarian carcinoma. Nature 474(7353):609–615
8. Hewitt SM, Badve SS, True LD (2012) Impact of preanalytic factors on the design and application of integral biomarkers for directing patient therapy. Clin Cancer Res 18:1524–1530
9. Zlobec I, Koelzer VH, Dawson H, Aurel Perren A, Lugli A et al (2013) Next-generation tissue microarray (ngTMA) increases the quality of biomarker studies: an example using CD3, CD8, and CD45RO in the tumor microenvironment of six different solid tumor types. J Transl Med 11:104–110
10. Zenobi R (2013) Single-cell mebabolomics: analytical and biological perspectives. Science 342:1201–1211
11. Vaught J, Henderson MK, Compton CC (2012) Biospecimens and biorepositories: from afterthought to science. Cancer Epidemiol Biomarkers Prev 21:253–255
12. US National Cancer Institute Biorepositories and Biospecimen Research Branch. http://www.biospecimens.cancer.gov. Accessed 15 Feb 2021

13. BBMRI (Biobanking and Biomolecular Resources Research Infrastructure). http://bbmri.eu/. Accessed 17 Dec 2013
14. Standardisation and improvement of generic pre-analytical tools and procedures for in-vitro diagnostics (SPIDIA). http://www.spidia.eu/. Accessed 15 Feb 2021
15. US National Cancer Institute Biorepositories and Biospecimen Research Branch, Biospecimen Research Network Symposia. http://biospecimens.cancer.gov/meeting/brnsymposium/. Accessed 15 Feb 2021
16. International Society for Biological and Environmental Repositories (ISBER) Biospecimen Science Working Group Publications. http://www.isber.org/?page=WGP. Accessed 15 Feb 2021
17. Engel KB, Moore HM (2011) Effects of preanalytical variables on the detection of proteins by immunohistochemistry in formalin-fixed, paraffin-embedded tissue. Arch Pathol Lab Med 135:537–543
18. Hewitt SM, Lewis FA, Cao Y et al (2008) Tissue handling and specimen preparation in surgical pathology: issues concerning the recovery of nucleic acids from formalin-fixed, paraffin-embedded tissue. Arch Pathol Lab Med 132:1929–1935
19. Wolff AC, Hammond ME, Schwartz JN et al (2007) American Society of Clinical Oncology/College of American Pathologists guideline recommendations for human epidermal growth factor receptor 2 testing in breast cancer. J Clin Oncol 25:118–145
20. ASCO–CAP HER2 Test Guideline Recommendations. Summary of guideline 2007 and 2013 recommendations. http://www.cap.org/apps/docs/committees/immunohistochemistry/summary_of_recommendations.pdf. Accessed 15 Feb 2021
21. Rollins G (2013) ASCO/CAP update HER2 testing guidelines. Clin Lab News. http://www.aacc.org/publications/cln/2013/december/Pages/HER2-Testing.aspx. Accessed 15 Feb 2021
22. Vaught J, Kelly A, Hewitt R (2009) A review of international biobanks and networks: success factors and key benchmarks. Biopreserv Biobank 7:143–150. https://doi.org/10.1089/bio.2010.0003
23. McShane LM, Altman DG, Sauerbrei W, et al.; for the Statistics Subcommittee of the NCI-EORTC Working Group on Cancer Diagnostics (2005) REporting recommendations for tumour MARKer prognostic studies (REMARK). Eur J Cancer. 41:1690–1696
24. Moore HM, Kelly A, Jewell SD et al (2011) Biospecimen reporting for improved study quality (BRISQ). Biopreserv Biobank 9:57–70. https://doi.org/10.1089/bio.2010.0036
25. Cheah S, Dee S, Cole A, Matzke L, O'Donoghue S, Watson PH (2012) An online tool for improving biospecimen data element reporting. Biopreserv Biobank 10:501–510. https://doi.org/10.1089/bio.2012.0033
26. National Cancer Institute Clinical Assay Development Program. https://cdp.cancer.gov/scientific_programs/pacct/cadp.htm. Accessed 15 Feb 2021
27. Williams PM, Lively TG, Jessup JM et al (2012) Bridging the gap: moving predictive and prognostic assays from research to clinical use. Clin Cancer Res 18:1531–1539
28. College of American Pathologists Biorepository Accreditation Program presentation. http://biospecimens.cancer.gov/meeting/brnsymposium/2012/docs/Day2_Denise_Driscoll_Presentation.pdf. Accessed 15 Feb 2021
29. International Society for Biological and Environmental Repositories (ISBER). http://www.isber.org. Accessed 15 Feb 2021
30. European, Middle Eastern and African Society for Biopreservation and Biobanking (ESBB). http://www.esbb.org. Accessed 15 Feb 2021
31. Rothman N, Hainaut P, Schulte P, et al., editors 2011 Molecular epidemiology: principles and practices. International Agency for Research on Cancer Publication Number 163, Lyon

Chapter 2
Biobank Design and Infrastructure: Biobank Engineering

Pasquale De Blasio and Ida Biunno

Abstract The availability of high-quality biological and environmental specimens for research purposes requires the development of standardized methods for collection, long-term storage, retrieval, and distribution of specimens. These practices require the implementation of a Certified Quality System specific for the Biobank (ISBER Biobank Proficiency Testing Program. https://www.isber.org/page/PTGI and BBMRI-ERIC Quality Management Services For Basic and Applied Research. https://www.bbmri-eric.eu/services/quality-management/).

In parallel, the biobank infrastructure needs to be designed and implemented (OECD Best Practice Guidelines for Biological Resource Centres. http://www.oecd-ilibrary.org/science-and-technology/oecd-best-practice-guidelines-for-biological-resource-centres_9789264128767-en; ISO/IEC 9001:2015 "Quality Management Systems requirements". https://www.iso.org/obp/ui/#iso:std:iso:9001:ed-5:v1:en; ISO 20387:2018, Biotechnology—Biobanking—General requirements for Biobanking. https://www.iso.org/standard/67888.html; and ISO/TC 212 "Clinical Laboratory Testing and in vitro diagnostic test systems". https://www.iso.org/committee/54916.html) with state-of-the-art technologies, and with the objective to be operative for periods up to 20–30 years. The commitment of the institution is critical to achieving this goal.

The technology which will be implemented (e.g., liquid nitrogen mechanical freezers, processing equipment, etc.) must be selected for present and future needs. Choices between manual and robotized equipment must be made, looking at future requirements, and considering the potential to improve the quality of the biobank. Backup systems (electrical and liquid nitrogen (LN_2)), remote back-up freezers, and sufficient space to expand are also mandatory for correct implementation and management of the biobank (OECD Best Practice Guidelines for Biological Resource Centres. http://www.oecd-ilibrary.org/science-and-technology/oecd-best-practice-guidelines-for-biological-resource-centres_9789264128767-en).

P. De Blasio (✉)
Integrated Systems Engineering, Brugherio, Italy
e-mail: pasquale.deblasio@isenet.it

I. Biunno
IRGB-CNR, Milan, Italy
e-mail: ida.biunno@isenet.it

P. Hainaut et al. (eds.), *Biobanking of Human Biospecimens*,
https://doi.org/10.1007/978-3-030-55901-4_2

In this chapter, we describe the most important aspects of biobank engineering, as complementary to, or integral to, the information included in the international guidelines for design and implementation of a state-of-the-art biobank.

Keywords Biobank engineering · ISO standard · Quality management system · Standard operating procedures · Biorepository accreditation program · Cryogenic room · LN_2 · Process laboratories

2.1 Introduction

The availability of high-quality biological and environmental specimens for research purposes requires the development of well-standardized methods of collection, processing, cryostorage, retrieval, and distribution of high-quality specimens. These practices require the implementation of a State-of-the-art infrastructure according to the International Guidelines [1–3], the definition of a Quality Management System (QMS) certified by ISO 9001:2015 [4] and were needed the accreditation of the Biobank QMS to CAP [5] (College of American Pathologists) and more recently by the new ISO 20387:2018 [6] specific for Biobanks.

The technologies and processes to be implemented (e.g., liquid nitrogen storage, mechanical freezers, processing equipment, etc.) should take into consideration present and future needs, looking at medium and long periods, according to the purpose/scope of the Biobank (e.g., Population, Disease, Animal, Environmental, Personalized Medicine, etc.).

Monitoring and Control Systems must be engineered to ensure the safety of the Biobank personnel and to guarantee the safety of the biospecimens stored by controlling the "cold chain." The infrastructure should have backup systems (electrical CO_2 and liquid nitrogen (LN_2)), remote storage and disaster recovery plan) in addition to sufficient space to expand and ensure medium-long time frame operability. Choices between manual and robotized equipment must be made, looking at future requirements, and considering the potential to improve the Biobank workflow and the quality of the biospecimens. The process laboratory should imply the Quality Control Procedures for all processes verified (if possible) by ISBER Assessment [7] and Proficiency [8] tools, and the SPIDIA self-assessment tool for molecular diagnostics to check pre-analytical workflows [9].

Management/Owners of the Biobank is fundamental for the success of the operation and its sustainability over time. Resources of the Biobank should be "structured" and trained in all aspects of Operation and Safety Procedure. The goal of the Biobank should be part of International Biobanking Networks (e.g., ISBER, ESBB, BBMRI, etc.) with the objective to distribute high-quality biospecimens and associated data to the Scientific Community.

2.2 Biobanking Engineering

Most of the information related to the construction and management of a Biobank are indicated in the guidelines prepared by major international biobanking societies (ISBER [3], NCI [2], BBMRI [14, 15], etc.) or international organizations (e.g., OECD [1], WHO [10, 11], etc.).

In addition, the International Standard Organization (ISO) has published the ISO 20387:2018 [6] "Biotechnology-Biobanking—General requirements for biobanking," to which all Biobanks should consider complying and be certified and/or accredited.

A Biobank should be engineered with state-of-the-art technologies taking into consideration the construction specificity for each of the following areas which are detailed in each specific chapter:

1. Cryogenic room (LN2 Distribution system; Cryogenic containers; etc.)
2. IT infrastructure (Monitoring and Control System; Laboratory Information Management System (LIMS))
3. Processing laboratories (Tissue, Cell and Molecular Biology, etc.)
4. Logistics and services (receiving and shipping services)

The Management of the Biobank should be formalized by a specific Quality Management System described in the following chapter.

2.3 Quality Management System (QMS)

A Quality Management System is a managerial tool that includes quality control and operational procedures like standard operating procedures (SOPs), to ensure consistent operations. The adoption of a QMS is a strategic decision for a Biobank since will improve its overall performance and provide a sound basis for sustainable developmental initiatives.

The potential benefits of implementing a "QMS" based on ISO 9001:2015 [4] are: (a) customer focus; (b) leadership; (c) engagement of people; (d) process approach; (e) continuous improvement; (f) evidence-based decision-making; and (g) relationship management.

This ISO 9001:2015 [4] International Standard promotes the adoption of a process approach when developing, implementing, and improving the effectiveness of a QMS, to enhance customer satisfaction by meeting customer requirements specifying general requirements for the competence, impartiality and consistent operation of biobanks including quality control requirements to ensure biological material and data collection of appropriate quality.

The new ISO 20387:2018 [6, 13, 17] standard specific for Biobanks is applicable to all organizations performing biobanking, including biobanking of biological material from multicellular organisms (e.g., human, animal, fungus, and plant) and microorganisms for research and development.

Biobank users, regulatory authorities, organizations and schemes using peer-assessment, accreditation bodies, and others can also use this document in confirming or recognizing the "**Competence of Biobanks.**"

The ISO 20387:2018 [6, 13, 17] Standards do not apply to biological material intended for food/feed production, laboratories undertaking analysis for food/feed production, and/or therapeutic use.

2.4 Structural Requirements of a Cryogenic Room

A cryogenic room is an infrastructure designed and built for storage at low temperatures, generally through the use of cryogenic fluids, of biological material for research and/or clinical use. A cryogenic room must have suitable and dedicated rooms, with characteristics adapted for specific functions. The equipment used must be adequate for the activity that will be carried out and in compliance with current safety regulations. The staff must be structured, qualified and dedicated to the cryogenic activities and trained for each specific task and under the direction of a Manager with specific experience with cryogenic substances (e.g., Liquid Nitrogen, CO_2, etc.). This Management role may be covered by the Head of the Biobank. Standard Operating Procedures (SOP's) for all cryogenic activities must be in place according to the QMS of the Biobank.

The design of the cryogenic room must guarantee:

- the safety of the people working in the cryogenic room
- the safety of the biological material cryo-stored
- the safety of the data (clinical, biological, and identification/traceability).

Particular attention must be given to Environmental Conditions and to possible new conditions caused by "climate changes" differently affecting various areas of the world, where heavy rain, floods, and/or earthquakes were rare or unusual in the past geological era. Every year we observe devastating tornados, sometimes related to hurricanes (e.g., the Katrina tornado outbreak across the eastern United States from August 29 to August 31, 2005, etc.) destroy cities and can affect biorepositories. This new reality must be taken into consideration when establishing a new biorepository infrastructure and defining a disaster plan. It is important therefore to look at the location of the biobank (examining the latest pattern of local disasters) and evaluate the risks of environmental conditions for the years ahead.

2.4.1 Definitions

- **Nitrogen (N_2)**: an inert, odorless, and colorless gas with a boiling point of 77.35 K (−195.8 °C).
- **Cryogenic fluid**: a fluid that boils at atmospheric pressure at temperatures below −73 °C.
- **Liquid nitrogen**: nitrogen is reduced to a liquid state by compression with a temperature of about −196 °C. It is part of the cryogenic fluids.
- **Liquid nitrogen storage tank**: cryogenic tank, complete with accessories required by the relevant regulations, consisting of two containers, one internal and one external, separated by an insulating cavity normally under vacuum. The cryogenic tank, normally placed in a suitable external environment, provides liquid nitrogen to the system and is the delivery point of the gas supplier.
- **Cryogenic container**: containers of variable dimensions containing nitrogen in liquid phase. Pressurized and non-pressurized containers can be distinguished.
- **Cryobiological container**: non-pressurized container of variable dimensions for short/medium/long-term nitrogen storage of biological samples. It is available in cryobiological containers with automatic and/or manual filling.
- **Programmable control rate freezer**: device used to gradually lower the freezing temperature of the biological samples.
- **Personal Protective Equipment (PPE)**: all the equipment worn and held by the worker in order to protect himself against any risk occurring during work activities. Risks related to personnel safety and/or health while at work, as well as any complement or accessory intended for this purpose.
- **Self-contained breathing apparatus**: device for breathing with air reserve in the case of low oxygen alarm.
- **Environmental oxygen detectors:** devices that continuously monitor the percentage of atmospheric oxygen inside the rooms, connected to an alarm system which alerts under-oxygenation in the room.
- **Aeraulic air treatment system**: set of all equipment, structures, accessories, and controls designed to ensure air quality maintaining specific microclimatic conditions. The definition includes air conditioning, thermo-ventilation, and ventilation.
- **Liquid nitrogen distribution system/cryogenic line**: pipelines that transfer liquid nitrogen from the external vessel to each cryogenic container. The line consists of a system of pipes that connect the main cryogenic vessel to the cryogenic container which does not need to be—insulated or vacuum insulated. The piping includes all necessary valves, fittings, and tools.
- **Safety valve**: automatic device whose function is to prevent that the pressure of a system containing liquids or gases can exceed a determined calibration and/or safety value.
- **Bursting discs**: safety device mounted on pressure vessels whose function is to prevent explosion or damage due to pressure build-up in a relatively short period of time.

2.4.2 *Identification and Characteristics of the Cryogenic Area*

The design and operation of the storage area (Cryogenic room) are very important, being the place where the biological material will be stored for long periods of time and where the safety of the biologicals and of operators must be guaranteed.

The cryogenic room must be of adequate size and have a location appropriate and designated for the specific purpose for which it will be used.

It is not recommended to handle and store liquid nitrogen in a local volume smaller than 20 m^3. Sufficient space must be provided for the handling of nitrogen containers, nitrogen samples, and personnel; it is advisable that the space of maneuvering is at least equal to the size of the largest cryogenic container. The distance between the nitrogen containers and the walls of the room should not be less than 30 cm and the distance between the nitrogen containers not less than 20 cm. It is also advisable to have a height of the rooms (net) not less than 2.70 m; in all cases, especially if the height is less than the recommended height, then it is recommended to furnish adequate ventilation systems able to maintain the percentage of oxygen at security levels.

The room must be physically isolated from other rooms or workplaces and must not be used as a passageway to access other locations. It should be dry, cool, well ventilated, and free of heat sources. It must be possible to view the interior of the cryobiology room through a window positioned on the door access or other viewing mode (e.g., glass walls). No other work must be carried out other than those processes provided for the management of liquid nitrogen and its use, nor should the room be used for the deposit of other material; however, it may be permitted to use the space for the positioning of freezers with CO_2 or nitrogen backup and for freezing biological samples with control rate freezers (Fig. 2.1a, b).

2.4.2.1 Access Door(s)

The access to the cryogenic room must be through an access door whose net size must be larger than the size of the largest containers contained in the location. Devices must be provided to prevent the spreading of gas in liquid or gaseous phase outside through the access door, which must also be provided with an opening toward the outside by means of a panic bar to allow rapid evacuation of personnel.

If the room has another access opening, it must also have the same access opening characteristics.

The access door must not be equipped with a spring closing device.

Usually, the access door is fitted with a visual device made of secure material which allows the room to be viewed from the outside (Fig. 2.2).

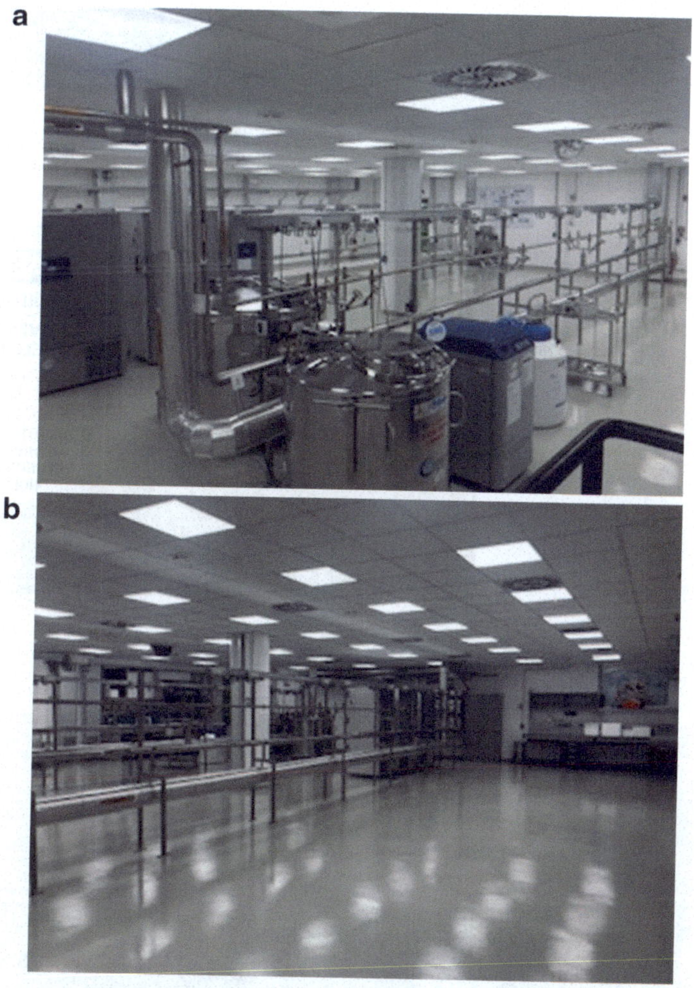

Fig. 2.1 (a) Cryo-room view 1 (b) Cryo-room view 2

2.4.2.2 Flooring and Walls

The room must be equipped with floors and walls (at least up to a height of 1.80), with waterproofing characteristics which can easily be sterilized. The floor and the cladding must be connected to each other in such a way as to avoid accumulation of dirt and dust and must be covered with a low-temperature resistant material easily maintained.

The cryogenic room floor must be covered with a special resin resistant to liquid nitrogen spills. The surface of the floor must also be very hard and strong in order to support the weight of the liquid nitrogen tanks and also very smooth in order to ease movements of the liquid nitrogen containers. The floor must not allow pouring liquid nitrogen into sewers or technical nets (Fig. 2.3).

Fig. 2.2 Access Door with windows and warning signs

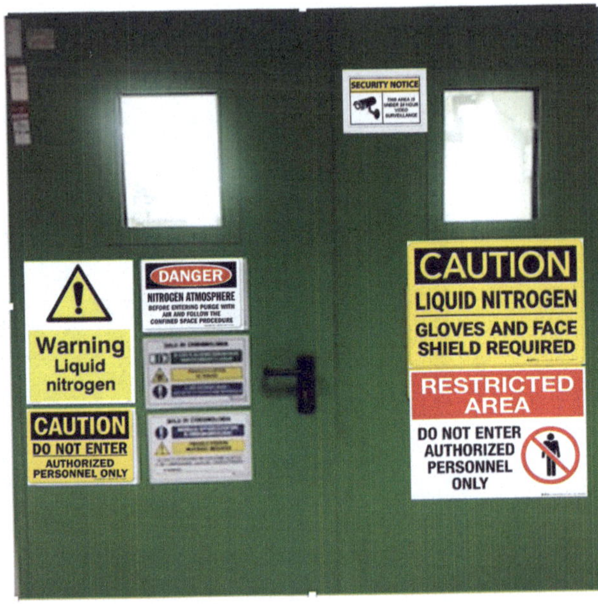
SECURITY NOTICE
DANGER
NITROGEN ATMOSPHERE
Warning
Liquid
nitrogen
CAUTION
DO NOT ENTER
AUTHORIZED
PERSONNEL ONLY
CAUTION
LIQUID NITROGEN
GLOVES AND FACE
SHIELD REQUIRED
RESTRICTED
AREA
DO NOT ENTER
AUTHORIZED
PERSONNEL
ONLY

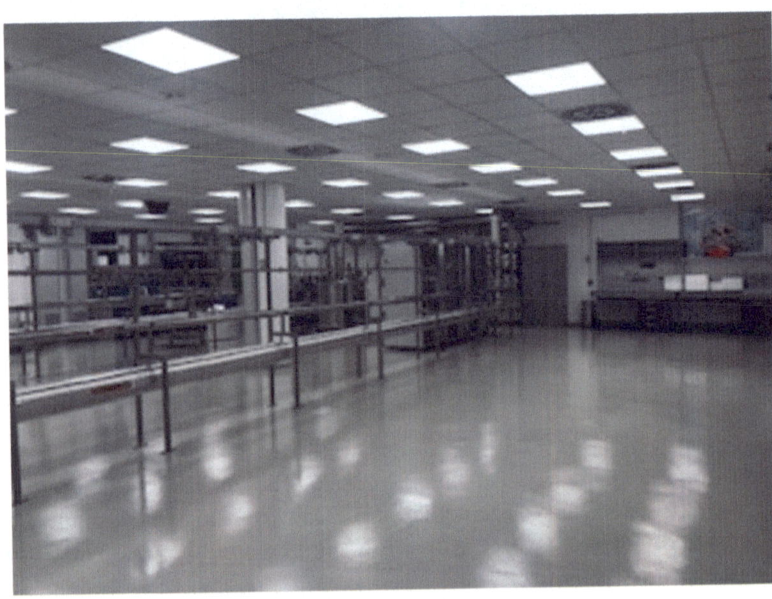

Fig. 2.3 Cryoroom Floor made with material resistent to LN2 spill

2.4.3 *Requirements for a Cryogenic Room*

The cryogenic room is classified as a hazardous area. Any spill of liquid nitrogen and/or liquid nitrogen vapor can cause clouds of low oxygen atmosphere, both being very dangerous for the personnel. Liquid nitrogen vapor, being heavier than air, accumulates in the area near the floor level, creating a cloud with low oxygen concentration.

2.4.3.1 Safety Systems

Monitor and Control System

Each cryogenic room must have a monitor and control system. The system must control the critical parameters of the cryogenic room (e.g., low oxygen levels, low level of liquid nitrogen in each container, low temperature in each mechanical freezer, environmental conditions such as temperature, humidity, and ventilation of the cryogenic room). Any of these conditions must signal an alarm to the authorized personnel, who will intervene 24/7 to analyze and fix the problem. Each alarm condition must also be recorded and discussed during the internal audits where preventive actions will be planned to avoid their recurrence. The monitoring and control system must record "continuously" the temperature of the LN2 containers and mechanical freezers, in order to follow freezing conditions over time of the biological material stored in each LN_2 container or ultra-low freezer (Fig. 2.4a, b).

The authorized personnel must be on call 24 h per day, 7 days per week in order to guarantee rapid and prompt intervention. The personnel authorized to work in the cryogenic room must be also trained to work with liquid nitrogen and to intervene in case of a low oxygen alarm condition (Fig. 2.5).

Access Control

Access to the cryogenic room must be controlled and limited exclusively to the authorized personnel. The cryobiological room must be equipped with a system for the monitoring and recording (history) of the accesses. A Standard Operating Procedure must be available which describes the terms and conditions for access to the cryogenic room of authorized personnel and external visitors under the responsibility of the Biobank Manager.

The personnel authorized to work in the cryogenic room must be qualified and trained to use an oxygen mask. This equipment must be placed outside of the cryogenic room and used by skilled personnel in case an operator is trapped in a low oxygen atmosphere area. Access to the cryogenic room is permitted only for two people at the same time. Both of them must carry a portable oxygen sensor. It is advisable that a third person will remain outside the cryoroom to intervene in case of emergency. If this precaution is not applicable, it is necessary to put in place

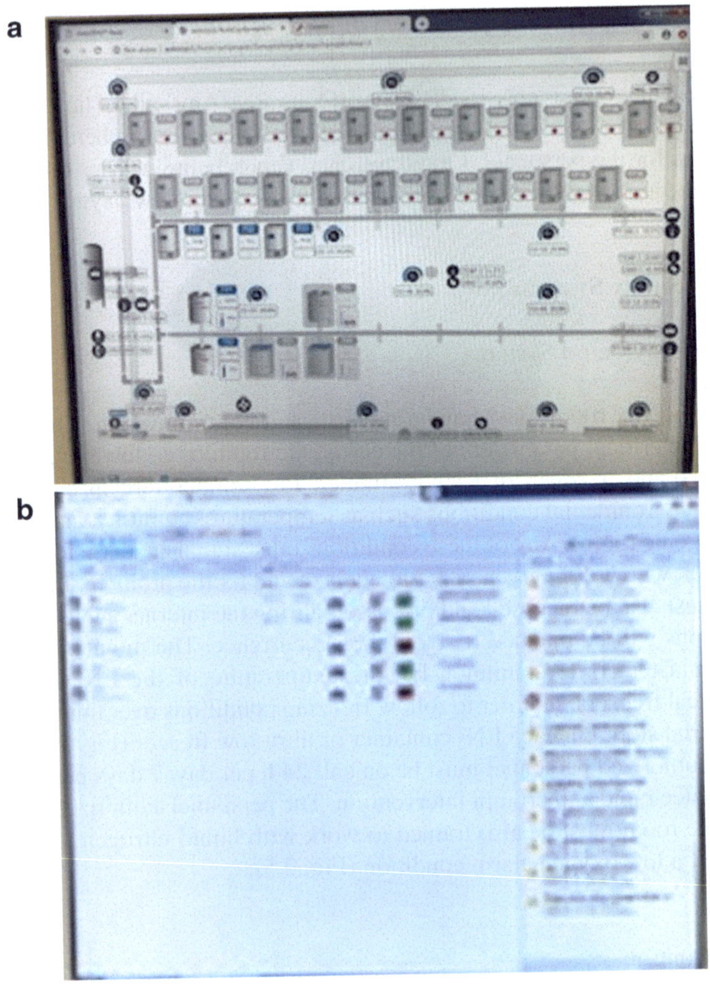

Fig. 2.4 (**a**) Monitoring and Alarm Systems Control Panel 1 (**b**) Monitoring and Alarm System Control Panel 2

alternative solutions that guarantee the safety of operators. Outside the cryogenic room must be an emergency kit consisting of self-contained breathing apparatus, preferably two-way (also to be assessed on the basis of risk assessment), gloves cryogenic, cryogenic apron, visor or goggles, and possibly cryogenic overshoes. These devices are located in a specially designed area identified. These devices must be periodically maintained and checked according to the specifications of the supplier (Fig. 2.6a, b).

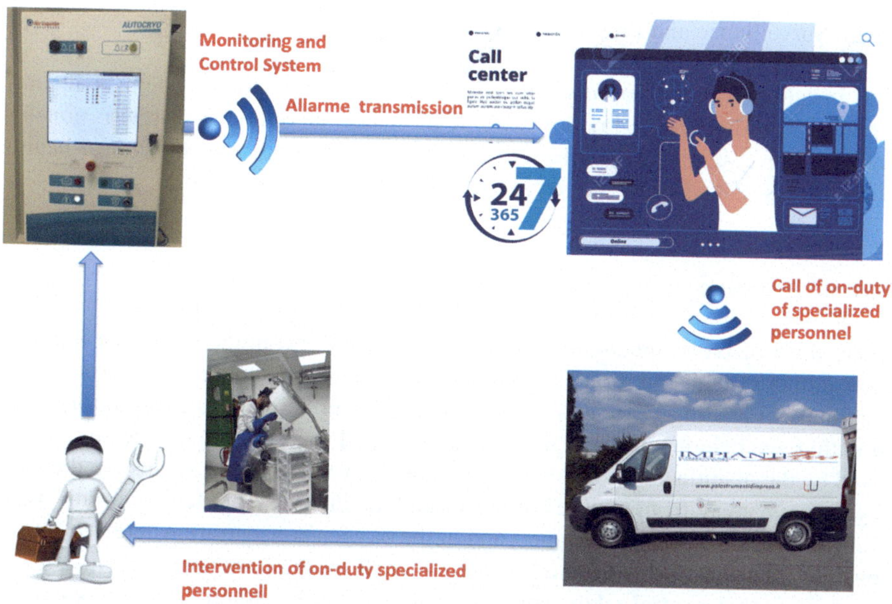
Monitoring and
Control System
Allarme transmission
Call
center
24
365
7
Call of on-duty
of specialized
personnel
Intervention of on-duty specialized
personnell

Fig. 2.5 Alarm system workflow

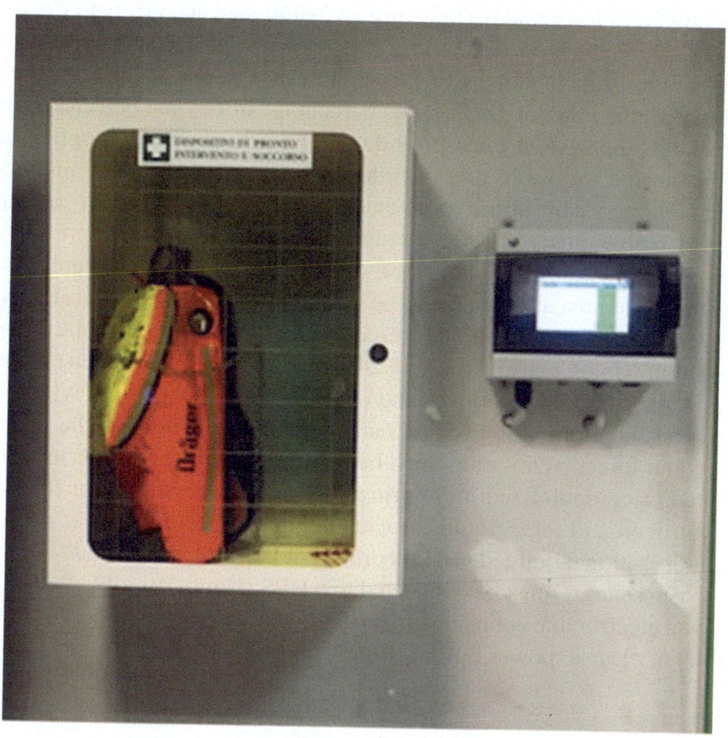

Fig. 2.6 Oxhygen Mask position outside of the Cryoroom

Video Surveillance and Presence Detection System

The installation of video surveillance and presence detection system is recommended according to the Privacy laws. If the video surveillance system is considered excessive, it is necessary to set up a procedure that prevents the risk of health emergencies related to the sub-oxygenation of the cryogenic room.

Oxygen Detection

There must be environmental oxygen detectors (sensors) in the room that monitor the continuous concentration of oxygen inside. These detectors must be placed at a height not exceeding 1.2 m and in any case at a lower height to the respiratory tract of authorized personnel. These detectors, calibrated according to maintenance indicated by the manufacturer, must be located in less ventilated areas, close to the passage points, away from sources of steam and air intakes. The detection unit must allow the visualization of the values and of the oxygen concentration detected by the sensor(s) and must be positioned outside the hall, in the immediate vicinity of the entrance so that control takes place in a safe area. It is essential that an adequate number of detectors defined according to the configuration and volume of the room and according to the type and characteristics of the sensor. It is recommended to install at least one detector for every 50 m^3. The detectors must comply with the relevant standard in force and periodically be maintained according to the supplier's instructions.

The system must have at least two alarm thresholds, one at the concentration of oxygen at **19%**, the other at **18%**. If the percentage of oxygen detected falls below these thresholds the system must provide for the activation of an optical-acoustic alarm either inside the room and outside. In addition, the alarm must activate a forced ventilation system in the room and, at reaching the 18% oxygen threshold, should also involve closure of the vacuum line root valve, where present and the interruption of supply of nitrogen in case of an automatic filling system. The forced ventilation system must also be able to be started manually by an operator. An alarm repetition (remote control) must be foreseen, at least for the second alarm threshold, or in a location (Call Centre) operative 24/7 that allows to warn the staff in charge and possibly the emergency services and/or to health care or directly with the operators. The acoustic alarm systems and visual surveillance systems, the operation of the probes, and forced ventilation must be controlled and verified periodically.

A manual or computerized monitoring system must be set up for following the levels of nitrogen and temperature of each container, according to a procedure or instruction operational defined. The recording of these monitors must be available.

The oxygen sensors must be connected to a UPS (Uninterruptible Power Supply) line and to an electric line connected to an emergency generator, in order to function during a major electric power failure (Fig. 2.7a, b).

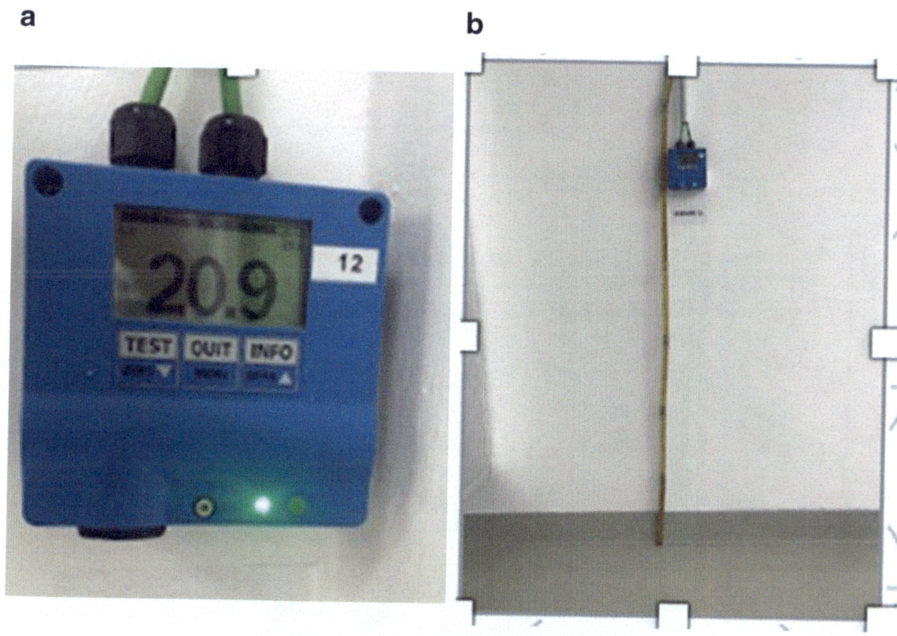

Fig. 2.7 (**a**) Oxygen sensor (**b**) Oxhygen sensor position

Ventilation and Environmental System

The cryogenic room must be equipped with an air treatment system able to control and maintain the temperature values between 18 and 25 °C to avoid condensation on the coldest parts of the cryogenic and ice deposition plant inside the storage tanks and humidity between 45–50% ± 5%, depending also on the seasonal period.

The ventilation system shall have an autonomous air intake and extraction system which need to ensure an adequate exchange of ambient air and avoid nitrogen accumulation. The ventilation system must be "full external air" type therefore without recirculation of the air taken from the environment and must ensure at least 6 air exchange/hour in "normal conditions" and 25 air exchange/hour (in any case not less than 20), in case of "alarm conditions."

It is of fundamental importance that the air intake takes place from above while the extraction takes place from below. The air extraction grille must be positioned preferably at a height of 10–15 cm from the floor. The mechanics of the system must be positioned in such a way as to prevent it from freezing in the event of abnormal leakage of nitrogen (Fig. 2.8a, b).

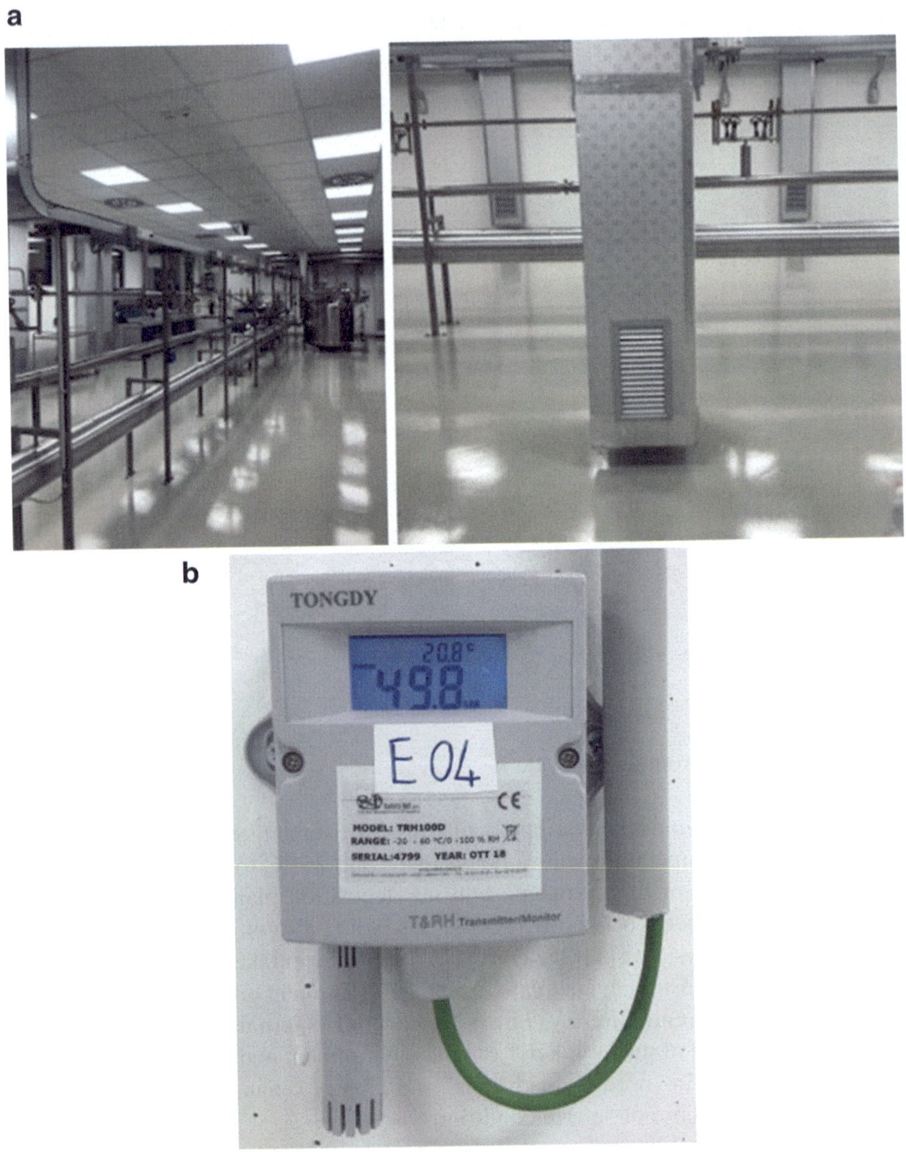

Fig. 2.8 (**a**) Cryo-room ventilation System Intake from top - Exhaust from Bottum (**b**) Temperature and Humidity sensor

Security Signs

At the entrance of the cryogenic room, signs must be displayed that indicate that the storage room is classified as dangerous: (1) sign of danger area: liquid nitrogen inside; possible low oxygen concentration; danger frostbite (2) sign requiring the wearing of personal protective equipment; (3) sign of warning: “In case of activation of the optical-acoustic alarm leave immediately the room and close the access door”; (4) prescription sign: “Inside of this room are permitted only operations of freezing and storage of biological material” (5) biohazard sign, etc. (Fig. 2.2).

Smoke Detection Systems

A fire detection system must be installed that can detect and report the presence of a fire inside the Biobank. A detection device smoke and fire are typically made up of electronic equipment that detects smoke and fire presence of smoke or variations in heat or the principle of fire. The anti-fire system must be remote-controlled and managed 24/7 (Fig. 2.9).

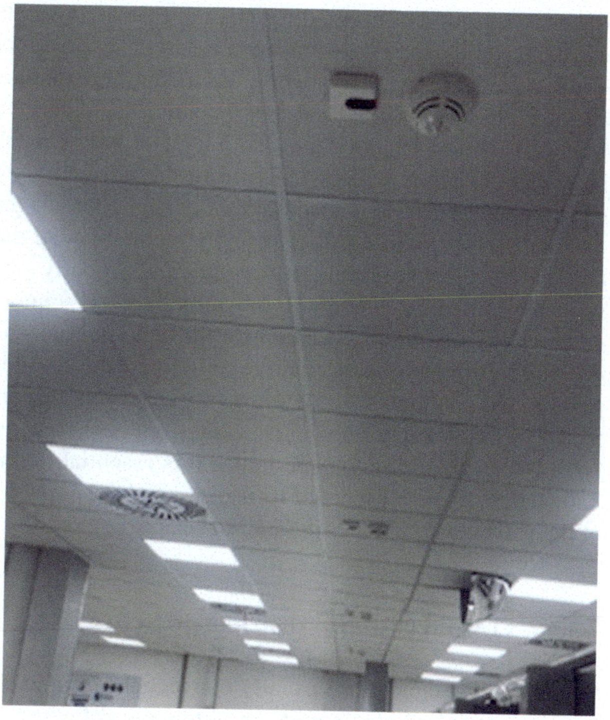

Fig. 2.9 Smoke sensorsr

Electrical and Lighting System

Natural and artificial lighting must comply with the National Electric Standard and regulations. An external switch must allow the internal artificial lighting to be switched on.

The power supply of the various types of equipment present in the cryogenic room must be insured, by adopting one or more general electrical panels, located outside the room, equipped with electrical power lines to guarantee separate lines for (a) Lights; (b) LN2 containers and/or mechanical freezers; (c) Other power appliances (video surveillance system and other accessories); (d) Uninterruptible Power Supply (UPS); (e) Emergency Generator; (f) Air treatment system; and (g) Oxygen monitoring system.

2.4.4 *Technological Features of a Cryogenic Room*

2.4.4.1 Storage Tanks and Liquid Nitrogen Supply

The liquid nitrogen distribution pipes must be vacuum pipes specifically designed for the purpose and must have safety valves that close automatically, in case of a low oxygen alarm in the cryogenic area, or in case of any malfunction or dangerous situation. Normally the liquid nitrogen reservoir is positioned outside the building as close as possible to the cryogenic room, and must be accessible by a trailer truck, and must have all safety features including the safety valve. The efficiency of the LN2 distribution system depends on the number of cryobiological containers, their size, their location, and distance from the nitrogen external tank. The LN_2 high-capacity tank must be placed outdoors, in an open-air fenced area with easy access to vehicles for refueling. It is strongly recommended that the tank is positioned in an area away from normal traffic routes and properly signed. The access to the tank must be limited exclusively to the authorized personnel. It is necessary to have an emergency stop button, located near the tank, in order to be able to stop the transfer of liquid nitrogen if needed. If the refilling of the cryogenic containers is done with pressurized containers, these must be placed in a dry and ventilated location, protected from atmospheric agents, away from heat sources, protected from fire risks. Even if the supplier owns the tanks, it is essential that the personnel has adequate knowledge of every aspect of its use system, and in particular the exact arrangement of the valves and switches in order to be able to close the tanks in case of emergency.

2.4.4.2 Liquid Nitrogen Distribution System

Cryogenic containers are usually connected to liquid nitrogen distribution system (vacuum stainless steel) with an automatic refueling system. The stainless steel pipes must be labeled to highlight the presence of liquid nitrogen and the direction of the flow. Inside the cryogenic room, connections must be provided on the vacuum line, including cryogenic and safety valves, conveyed to the outside, for the connection of the cryogenic containers. The maximum pressure of the liquid nitrogen inside the pipes, must not exceed the maximum pressure indicated by the manufacturer of the cryogenic containers. The line must also be equipped with safety devices (safety valves or rupture disks) as described in the technical specifications to avoid any risk of explosion. In the case of insulated or vacuum distribution lines of considerable length, it should be equipped with an open-air vent valve (vent valve) position in the bottom of the line with external coating, for the removal of nitrogen vapors during the cooling of the line itself. All manual valves used on the line must be suitable for cryogenic applications. Distribution lines must not constitute a source of danger and must be prevented from being the source of formation of hazardous gas atmospheres as a result of leaks and ruptures, which can cause leakage and stagnation. They must be inspectable. At the beginning of the line must be installed a by-pass system with a solenoid valve. A planimetric representation of the piping system must be available with highlighting of the interception systems (Fig. 2.10a, b).

2.4.5 *Equipment*

2.4.5.1 Cryogenic Containers

The cryobiological container is a type of equipment capable of storing biological samples under controlled temperature. Various types of cryobiological containers are available: Liquid Nitrogen Tanks (−196 °C); Liquid Nitrogen Vapor Tanks (−80 °C, −155 °C); Mechanical Ultra-Low Freezers (−80 °C, −150 °C); Cold Rooms (from −20 to −80 °C); Automatic Storage Rooms (−80 °C); Liquid Nitrogen Vapor Freezers (−155 °C); etc.

The choice of the type of container must be made according to the characteristics of the biological material to be cryopreserved, the number of samples to be stored, and the characteristics of the cryogenic room and liquid nitrogen refueling system.

Liquid Nitrogen (LN_2) Containers

Biobanks should have a number of cryogenic containers, compatible with the structural characteristics of the room and connected to an automatic LN_2 filling system. The number of LN_2 containers must be compatible with the design specifications of the distribution system and the presence of containers in series. Cryogenic containers must be subject to control in accordance with the current standard and according to a specific maintenance plan. The containers must be equipped with racks according to the type and dimensions of the vessel (bags, cryo box, cryotubes, etc.) that hold the biosamples, allowing adequate protection and traceability during storage

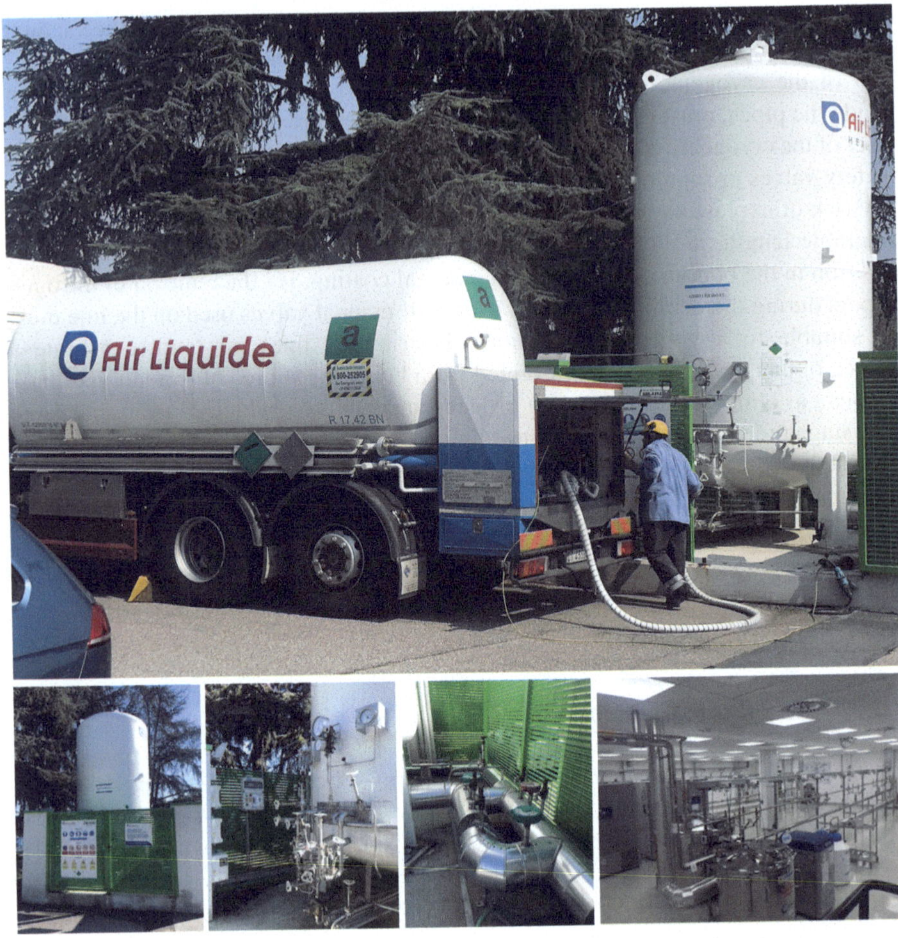

Fig. 2.10 Liquid Nitrogen external vessel

and adequate protection of the samples during storage. Manual or automatic detection and recording systems must be provided, nitrogen levels and temperature of each cryobiological container. In both cases, such monitoring must be continuous and the storage/recording of data at the maximum every 4 h. The definition of container filling levels and values of the storage temperature must be subject to validation protocols, for the maintenance of the morphological, biological, and functional characteristics of the samples preserved. The alarm systems must be set up in case of deviation of the values measured with respect to the defined standard. Smaller tanks that are not connected to an automatic refueling system are subjected to manual control as specified by the relevant SOPs.

Manual Filling of Cryobiological Containers

In case of manual filling of liquid nitrogen, it is necessary that the container is empty and contains only nitrogen, not water or other cryogenic liquids. It is possible to use a funnel to transfer the liquid into a smaller container. It is recommended to use a transfer tube to extract the liquid or a pressure tapping system. Manual filling operations must be carried out in the cryogenic room or in any case in an adjacent room with the same security features. At least two operators must be present in the room, use PPE to avoid eyes and skin to get in contact with liquid nitrogen, cold tubes, or cold gas.

Handling of Cryogenic Containers

In the event that it is necessary to move cryogenic containers within the structure, attention must always be paid to unintentional releases of emissions of cold vapors from the containers, which may cause progressive gas accumulation in the environment by reducing the oxygen content of the air. If the move of the container requires elevator lifts, it is necessary that the containers, in particular for those of considerable capacity, are moved in the absence of personnel. Narrow and closed lift can quickly saturate creating serious danger to personnel. When moving the container use the appropriate handles or trolleys. Do not attempt to lift the container by yourself, but possibly get some help from a second operator. The transport container must be equipped with a safe gripping system and a suitable lid.

2.4.5.2 Mechanical Ultra-Low Freezers (−80 °C)

The Biobank shall have a number of Mechanical Ultra-Low freezers, compatible with the structural characteristics of the room itself and connected to an automatic LN_2 or CO_2 backup system. The number of Mechanical Ultra-Low freezers must be compatible with the design specifications of Electric Power; Ventilation Systems; and the LN_2 or CO_2 backup system. If the Ultra-Low Freezer does not have either a LN_2 or CO_2 backup system, they must be connected to the Emergency Generator. The Ultra-Low Freezers must be subject-specific maintenance plan. The characteristics of these Ultra-Low Freezers, how to use them, and their maintenance must be specified in the manual of use and maintenance of every single device. The Ultra-Low Freezer must be equipped with racks according to the type and dimension of the container (bags, cry box, cryotubes, etc.) in which the biosample is stored, allowing adequate protection and traceability of the samples during storage. Manual or automatic detection and recording of the temperature of each Ultra-Low Freezer must be provided and recorded at least every 4 h. The Ultra-Low Freezers and values of the storage temperature must be subject to validation protocols according to the morphological, biological, and functional characteristics of the samples preserved. Alarm systems must be set up in case of deviation of the values measured with respect to the defined standard.

Check and cleaning procedures for air filters and ice formation inside of the doors of the freezers must be part of the maintenance plan.

2.4.5.3 Automatic Storage Systems (−80 °C, LN_2 Vapor −155 °C)

Biobanking storage technology evolved in the last 10–15 years with the development of several automatic storage systems which improve traceability, faster and precise storage/towing of biosample; steady temperature over time; space reduction, etc.

Installing Automatic Storage Systems requires an overall improvement of the Biobank design (structural characteristics, logistics, electric power, backup systems, monitoring and control systems, etc.) and needs to make significant advancement of the Biobank workflow, which requires significant effort in interfacing the Biobanking LIMS with Automatic Storing Systems software.

Automatic Storing Systems are suitable for Large Biobanks where management and distribution of a large number of biosample, or for Specialized Biobanks (e.g., Tissue Bank Stem Cell Banks, etc.) where traceability and steady temperature over time is fundamental. In these cases, smaller Automatic systems are suggested (Fig. 2.11a–c).

2.4.5.4 Cold Chain Monitoring and Control

The cold chain must be monitored and controlled 24/7 and recorded by the Monitoring and Control system. In particular, the temperature of all Liquid Nitrogen Containers and the Ultra-Low Freezers should be controlled with two independent temperature control sensors so that if one temperature sensor brakes, the other loop is monitoring the temperature (Fig. 2.12).

2.4.6 Personal Protection Equipments (PPE)

PPE must be used when risks cannot be avoided or sufficiently reduced by technical prevention measures. Personnel must use these devices, take care of them without making changes, reporting any defects or inconveniences encountered. The use of some PPE is required for training and education purposes. Each PPE must be accompanied by the required documents (declaration of conformity by the manufacturer, CE marking, information note issued by the manufacturer). The Liquid Nitrogen Safety Data Sheet provides an essential indication of PPE that must be used when handling liquid nitrogen. Likewise, the user and maintenance manual for the purchased equipment specifying which PPE is required. For the entire time, all operators are obliged to wear the PPE when handling liquid nitrogen.

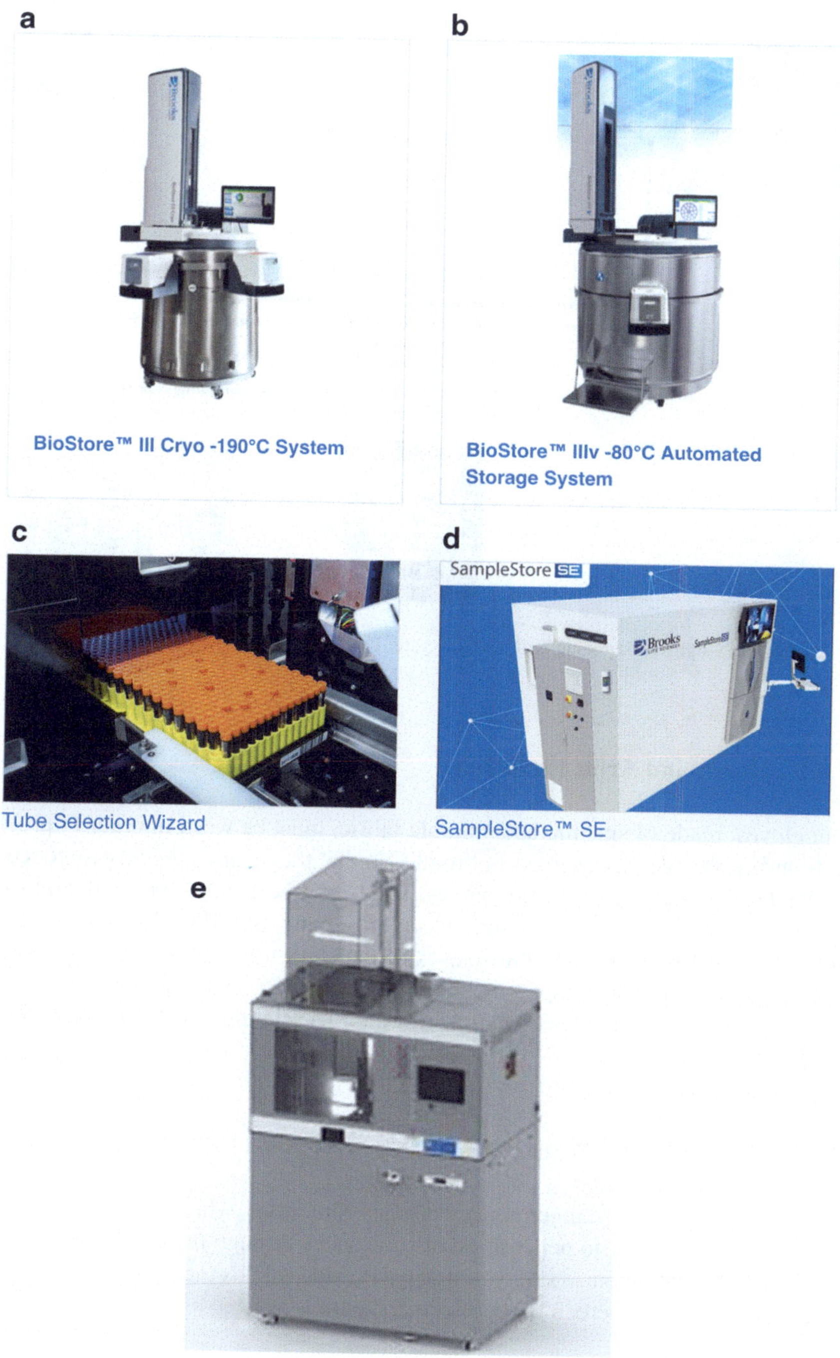

Fig. 2.11 (**a**) 196°C Robotised Cryogenic Container (Brooks Biostore) (**b**) 80°C Robotised Cryogenic Cotainer (Brooks Biosotre) (**c**) Cryovilas loading system for Storing Room (**d**) Automatic -80°C Storing room (Brooks SampleStore) (**e**) 196°C Robotised Freezer (Angelantoni SmartFreezer)

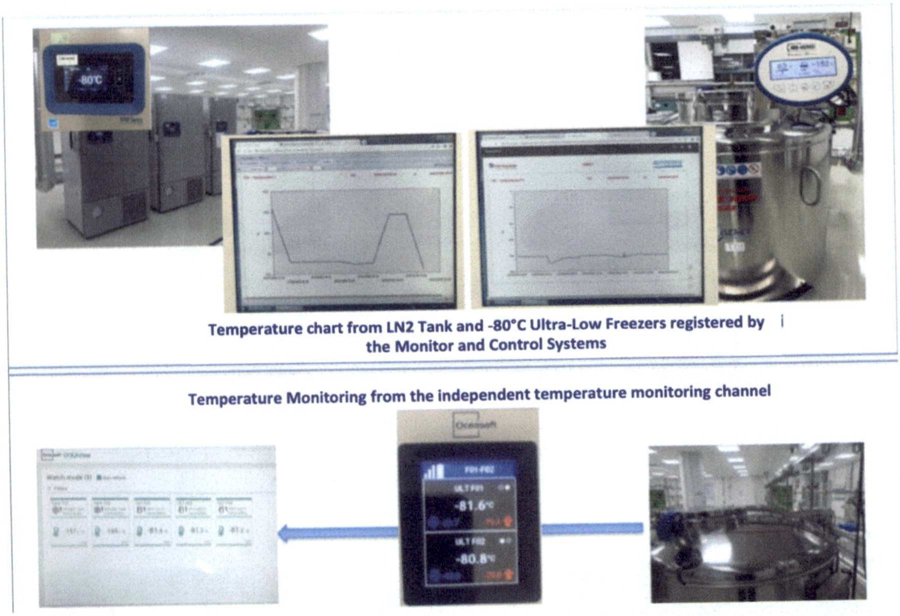

Fig. 2.12 Cold Chaim monitoring and control system

2.4.6.1 Hands and Arms Protection

Long gloves, made of specific and suitable fabric, must be worn in order to protect hands and arms. The gloves must fit broadly so that they can be quickly removed in case the liquid enters inside of the gloves. They must be checked before being used and inspected for damage or contamination (cuts, punctures, discolored spots, etc.). The gloves must be worn over the sleeves of the shirt, to avoid that drops of liquid fall on the shirt; moreover, they must be removed before resuming any other activity. The type of gloves and specifications for their use should in any case be detailed in a specific SOP.

2.4.6.2 Eyes and Face Protection

In case of particularly dangerous operations, situations which may give rise to splashes or, in any case, to penetration of substances through the eyes or the skin of the face, it is essential to use safety goggles with side shields (according to EN 166), better a visor or facial screen that protects the entire face.

2.4.6.3 Body Protection

For precaution, always wear trousers on the outside of boots or shoes. Generally, sandals or other **open-toed shoes are prohibited**. For special processing, including manual topping, which involves the exposure of the whole body at very low temperatures, protective aprons may be used or, in cases where more problematic, specific protection suits or gowns. It is strongly recommended to use cryogenic overshoes during manual filling operations, especially for small containers. Wear overalls or gowns, preferably without pockets.

2.4.7 Rules of Conduct

2.4.7.1 General Rules of Conduct which Must Be Adopted in a Cryogenic Room

Activities involving cryogenic fluids must be reserved only for those who have received adequate information and training on the correct procedures to be followed. All operations must be carried out according to SOP.

2.4.7.2 Specific Rules to Be Adopted in a Cryogenic Room

Below is a non-exhaustive list of specific behavioral norms of prevention:

- Always handle liquid nitrogen with utmost caution.
- Keep the container open for as short time as possible to avoid the danger of condensation and gas formation.
- Do not touch pipes and containers containing liquid nitrogen without PPI. There is a danger of skin burn.
- Do not pour unused liquid nitrogen into drains or on the floor; use only hot water to release frozen valves.
- Wear suitable PPE.
- Collect long hair behind the back of the neck.
- Always keep at a safe distance from boiling or splashing nitrogen and gas.
- It is advisable to use high or sufficiently closed shoes.
- When handling liquids in open containers take care not to spill them. Always wear trousers on the outside of the shoes.
- Always carry out the filling operations of a container or immersion of uncooled objects in the liquid in order to minimize boiling and splashes.
- Always use pliers with a secure grip to submerge or pull out objects immersed in cryogenic fluid, never use the hands.

- Avoid filling the containers beyond the safety level; excess liquid increases the evaporation rate and the danger of overflow during transport.
- To transfer full containers always use appropriate means (e.g., trolleys) and do not accompany them in the lift.
- Always remember that objects normally soft and foldable at room temperature environment become extremely hard and fragile at the temperature of these liquids.
- Avoid working alone during activities involving the use and/or the use of the liquid handling of liquid nitrogen.
- Warn colleagues before carrying out any operation particularly dangerous.
- Do not approach areas where hazardous operations are carried out if it is unnecessary.
- Respect all safety signs.
- Do not keep in the cryobiological room what is not strictly necessary for carrying out the activities (e.g., personal effects) and in particular bulky material or easily combustible.
- Do not use tubes to measure the level of liquid nitrogen (chimney effect).

2.4.7.3 Emergency Procedures

The availability of emergency operating procedures on possible expected accidental events is an indispensable protection system against associated risks on the use of cryogenic fluids; these procedures must be available and known by all workers.

To prevent emergency situations or allow problems to be resolved quickly it is essential to be able to recognize the signals that precede a failure in the system of containment. These can be:

- High pressures are indicated on the control pressure gauge.
- Unexpected frost formation on the containment system.
- Poor or abnormal venting in the containment system.
- Alarms indicating low oxygen levels in the work area.
- Unusual noise or absence of normal venting noise.

The typical signals of the release of a large amount of vapors due to evaporation of the cryogenic fluid are an increase in background noise and the formation of a plume of white fog. In this case, although the danger of under-oxygenation especially in poorly ventilated premises is never to be overlooked, generally the most harmful event probable is contact with gas or liquid at very low temperature with the consequences previously mentioned. In the event that the release is not large, for example, from a dewer of small size, it may be sufficient to transport the container outdoors and let the vapors escape into the atmosphere.

2.4.8 Information and Training

The Management of the Biobank, in collaboration with the Quality and Safety officers, has the obligation to provide adequate training for all operators working in the cryogenic room, including students, trainees, scholarship holders, guests, and other unstructured personnel. Training must be given in relation to the activities carried out, and the objective is to inform and train everyone on aspects such as risks related to the workplace and tasks; the possible damage resulting from the use of dangerous equipment or substances without due precautions; the prevention and protection measures to be implemented in each specific situation; fire-fighting measures and escape routes; emergency plan; and how to ensure the correct application of prevention and protection measures by all visitors to the cryogenic room itself.

2.5 Remote Storage

It is advisable that for renewable biospecimens (master and working cell lines, etc.) a biobank stores part of the stock (e.g., duplicates) in three different locations. (e.g., if the Biobanks generates 20 vials of one cell line, will store 12 vials in one cryogenic container; 4 vials in different containers in the Biobank; and the rest of the stock in a different accredited Biobank located 20–30 km away from the main location).

The Biobank can also be a reference to other Biobanks which will have the same needs.

2.6 Disaster Plan

A very important requirement for a Biobank is to establish a "disaster plan," which defines the actions to put in place in case of an unexpected "major disaster" (power failure, fire, flood, earthquake, etc.).

The disaster plan should consider the following aspects:

- ***Risk assessment of the Biobank Infrastructure*** for liquid nitrogen supply, electric power supply (also considering the emergency generators loads), environmental adverse events (historical statistics for floods, earthquakes, airplane disaster, etc.).
- ***Partner with a "Certified" or "Accredited" Biobank for support in case of a major disaster***. The choice of the partner biobank is very important and should follow a risk analysis looking at the following factors: (a) structured and certified biobanking infrastructure; (b) availability of free space to accommodate, in case

of major disaster, additional LN_2 containers and −80° Ultra-Low Freezers to be relocated from the original biobank; (c) sufficient liquid nitrogen and electric power supply; (d) low risk for environmental factors (flood, earthquake, tornados, etc.); (e) Biobanking LIMS for traceability; and (f) other factors.

- ***Agreements with specialized movers*** that have adequate equipment (e.g., trucks with electric supply), in order to have the possibility to refill the LN_2 containers and electric supply for the −80 °C ultra-low freezers during the transport of the cryogenic containers from one biobank to the other. It is also important to have the proper vehicle and transport authorization to transport tanks full of liquid nitrogen, etc.
- ***Understanding of local regulations to transport liquid nitrogen containers.*** Discuss and plan with local authorities with respect to the rules and regulations to follow during the move.
- ***For new Biobanking infrastructures***. Assess the local risks as indicated above and consider infrastructure solutions (e.g., building constructed to be earthquake-proof, cryogenic room located on the first floor, limit damage in case of a major adverse event such as basement flooding).

2.7 Process Laboratories

A Biobank is also characterized by the types and quality of the process/service able to perform. The process laboratories can be part of the Biobank as service unit, or part of the Hospital/Research Center where the Biobank is located.

The Process Laboratories are important to guarantee the highest quality of the biospecimen stored and distributed but must also be used to develop new procedures and standards to improve the quality of the biological material and shared with the Biobanking scientific community.

The types of Services and Laboratories can be identified according to their specialities:

- **Tissue process Laboratory:** dedicated to store frozen tissues (deep freezing technology) which will be stored in mechanical freezers at −80 °C.
- **Molecular Biology Laboratories**: dedicated to the quality control of the biomaterial, for example, nucleic acid purifications (DNA, RNA, microRNA) in addition to proteins that can be stored in mechanical freezers at −80 °C.
- **Cell Biology Laboratories**: dedicated to the establishment and immortalization of primary cell lines, eventually stored in LN_2 liquid at −196 °C or − 155 °C in LN_2 vapor tanks.
- Depending on the type and focus, the Biobank can have additional process and service laboratories such as:
- **Sequencing Facility**, usually for human biobanks or personalized medicine applications.

- **Tissue Microarray Core facility**, for tissue banks, which also store pathology archives, usually comprising paraffin-embedded tissues.
- **Other Core Facilities/Services complementing the "omics" platforms**.
- **Induced reprogramming adult stem cells and quality control Core facility**.

- The laboratories associated with biobanks are important for the processing of biological materials (such as whole blood) into derivatives such as buffy coats, plasma, cell lines, and nucleic acids. Laboratories are also involved in performing the quality control procedures in order to guarantee the integrity of the biological material stored and distributed and are also very important for offering services to the scientific community which may contribute to the recovery of costs of the Biobank operations.

In addition, considering the technological and scientific advancements of "Biobanking Science" the Biobanks shift their focus toward Personalized Medicine; Regenerative Medicine; Stem Cells and iPS; and most recently toward the generation and banking of 3D Organoids/Spheroids, which are used by the pharmaceutical industry for drug discovery research.

These shifts will require a change in the skills of the personnel of the Biobank and an expansion of the quality control procedures which will be used to characterize the biological material distributed.

The access to the laboratory must be controlled (with badge or other systems) and registered. Visits inside the laboratories should be discouraged. One solution, to avoid visitors entering inside the process areas, is to build the laboratory with large windows, and build corridors in the perimeter of the laboratories in order for visitors to have the possibility to view the activities in the process areas without entering them.

All the critical instruments should be connected to the electric power emergency line and/or to a UPS (Uninterruptible Power Supply) line.

2.8 Biobank IT Infrastructure

The IT infrastructure is one of the most important investments for a Biobank but is frequently overlooked and underestimated.

The choice of the Biobank Management Information System (LIMS) is not trivial (homemade or commercially available) and can be a very important part of the budget for the implementation of the Biobank and its efficient operation. It is important not to underestimate the effort of implementing the LIMS and the improvements that will be required during the years of the operation of the Biobank.

One other important aspect is the investment and effort required to store the data associated with the biospecimen, which are increasing exponentially considering the requirements of associates genetic data (e.g., sequencing data) and/or pathology images (which require large storage facilities). Backup and safety measures must also be planned and implemented.

It is also important to verify the risks and opportunities for the new technology (such as cloud computing) available today which will be improved and be used on a widespread basis in the near future.

The LIMS should have the capability to manage each step of the biospecimen life cycle including the administrative and financial aspects, which are important for the sustainability of the BRC.

The Biobanking LIMS must be able to manage the following aspects:

2.8.1 Clinical Data Management Information System

It is well known that biospecimens with associated high-quality clinical data are of great value and that biospecimens with no associated clinical data are generally less valuable. Therefore, the LIMS which will be implemented must be able to capture and manage clinical data, which needs to be associated with the biospecimen. This is not a trivial task, since the clinical data are usually stored in different sources (paper records, spreadsheets, clinical databases, etc.), often with different annotations/classification methods for the same disease.

The Biobank coordination center should define a minimum data set to be associated with each type of biospecimen and disease, in order to define a standardized LIMS module where the operators can upload the clinical data associated with the biospecimen in the correct format. Automated forms of data transfer are also possible and dependent on the organization of the collection site database and the relationship with the Biobank.

Biobank Management Information System (LIMS) should have the capability to track each phase of the biospecimen life cycle, from collection to distribution:

- **Biospecimen collection** (at donor collection site). The technician, at the collection site (usually a trained nurse), following specific SOPs, will obtain from the patient or donor minimum data set of clinical data and will place the biospecimens in bar-coded container (cryotubes, tissue cassette, etc.) which after being scanned will be up-loaded in a specific web page in the Biobank LIMS. After the biospecimen containers will be packaged and shipped to the Biobank site according to the specific SOP.
- The system should also have a specific section where to insert information relative to the shipping kit and the courier's tracking number. The LIMS will follow the shipment and send an email to the central biorepository with the information of the shipment.
- **Accessioning**. Upon arrival, the shipping kit will be accepted by a dedicated operator, who will upload the bar codes of the material received. The LIMS will check automatically if the biospecimens shipped are the same as the biospecimens received and generate an acceptance report or a rejection report in the event of a discrepancy. On the acceptance report, there is information such as shipping

date and time, high and low temperatures during the shipment, and delays at customs.
- According to requirements of the accessioning SOP for the specific project, which specify the intended use of each biospecimen collected, the tubes/containers will be transferred to the:
  - **Cryostorage room,** if the biomaterial received (e.g., frozen tissue, plasma, urine, PaxGene, etc.) does not need to be processed.
  - **Pathology Archive,** if the paraffin-embedded tissue blocks need to be archived.
  - **Molecular Biology Laboratory,** if the biological material needs to be processed (e.g., DNA purification from whole blood, saliva, etc.)
  - **Cell Biology Laboratory**, if the biological material needs to be processed for the establishment of primary or immortalized cell lines.
  - **Other destinations**, according to the relevant SOPS.
- **Processing of Biological material**. Each process for biological material must be performed according to a specific SOP. Each SOP will describe, for each biological material derived, the quality control or characterization data which must be uploaded into specific webpages available on the LIMS.
- It must be possible at each moment to track and verify a single process, progress, and any other problems. The LIMS will also periodically produce statistics (average time for each process, problems, etc.), which are to be discussed during the internal audits and generate corrective actions.
- **Inventory Management System.** The LIMS must incorporate an "Inventory Management System" to manage and track (via bar codes, radio frequency identification (RFID), or other identification methods) the biospecimen from the time of collection to the generation of derivatives (as a result of processing), to the final location storage container (LN_2 or Ultra-Low Freezer), minimizing the possibility of errors.
- **Storage facility**. The biological material can be stored at different temperatures (−196 °C in LN_2 Liquid Container; −155 °C in LN_2 Vapor Container; −80 °C Ultra-Low Freezer, −40 °C, −20 °C, +4 °C, and room temperature). The inventory system (embedded in the LIMS System) should guarantee the tracking of each biospecimen aliquot in its storage location. In some cases, for the same batch of samples different aliquots could be stored in different locations.
- The LIMS should also be interfaced with the monitor and control system in order to record alarm and storage conditions which must be associated with each specimen stored over time.
- **Quality Control**. Specific efforts must be dedicated to record the quality control data associated with each biospecimen stored and/or retrieved. Quality control data are not only the result of specific procedures (e.g., cell line viability, 260/280 nm ratio for DNA purity, etc.) but also the temperature of storage over time, and pre-analytical data if available. Quality Control reports should always

be available (via web) and accompany the biospecimen when distributed. In some cases, the QC reports are transmitted in the datasheet when the biospecimen is shared/distributed.

- **Distribution**. The possibility to distribute "high quality" biological material makes the difference between a Biobank and a Repository. The LIMS plays a very important role in tracking all phases of the distribution process, which starts with the request, authorization, retrieval of biomaterial, shipping, and invoicing. These administrative functions are very important for the sustainability of the Biobank.
- **The LIMS system should implement the following online functions**:
  - **Web-catalog**, with the list of the biomaterials stored and associated clinical data ready for distribution.
  - **Browse function of the web-catalog**, with the possibility to filter the biospecimen types and access the data (clinical and biological data) associated with the biospecimen.
  - **Requesting biospecimens**. This includes the possibility of accessing a web browser which will enable the researcher to browse for several parameters: demographic data (name, institution, etc.); informed consent (yes/no); clinical data (disease, follow-up, etc.); biological data (QC parameters); and number of biospecimens available. After the identification of the biospecimens needed, the researcher can fill a specific webpage (where it will be possible to upload the list of biospecimens needed) and fill in additional information such as name and institution information, abstract of the scientific project with a statement of the intended use of the biospecimens.
  - **Approval process:** This should also be managed online, where on a specific webpage the custodian of the biospecimens can follow the number of pending requests, can approve requests, or can ask for more information from the requester concerning the project and intended use, or can deny the authorization. At the same time, the requester and the biorepository manager can follow the approval process. After approval, the LIMS will send a work order to the biorepository with the authorization to retrieve and ship the material to the requester, according to conditions specified by the Material Transfer Agreement (MTA) (Fig. 2.13a, b).

2.9 Logistics and Services

The logistics and services units are as important as the other units since they keep the Biobank in functional order. In the following, there is a list of service units which may be part of the Biobank, according to its specific mission [16]:

1. **Collection Kit preparation**. Each project will have its specific collection needs, which requires the design of a specific collection kit. Usually, the collection kit includes (1) the appropriate collection vessel (e.g., Vacutainer for blood) with

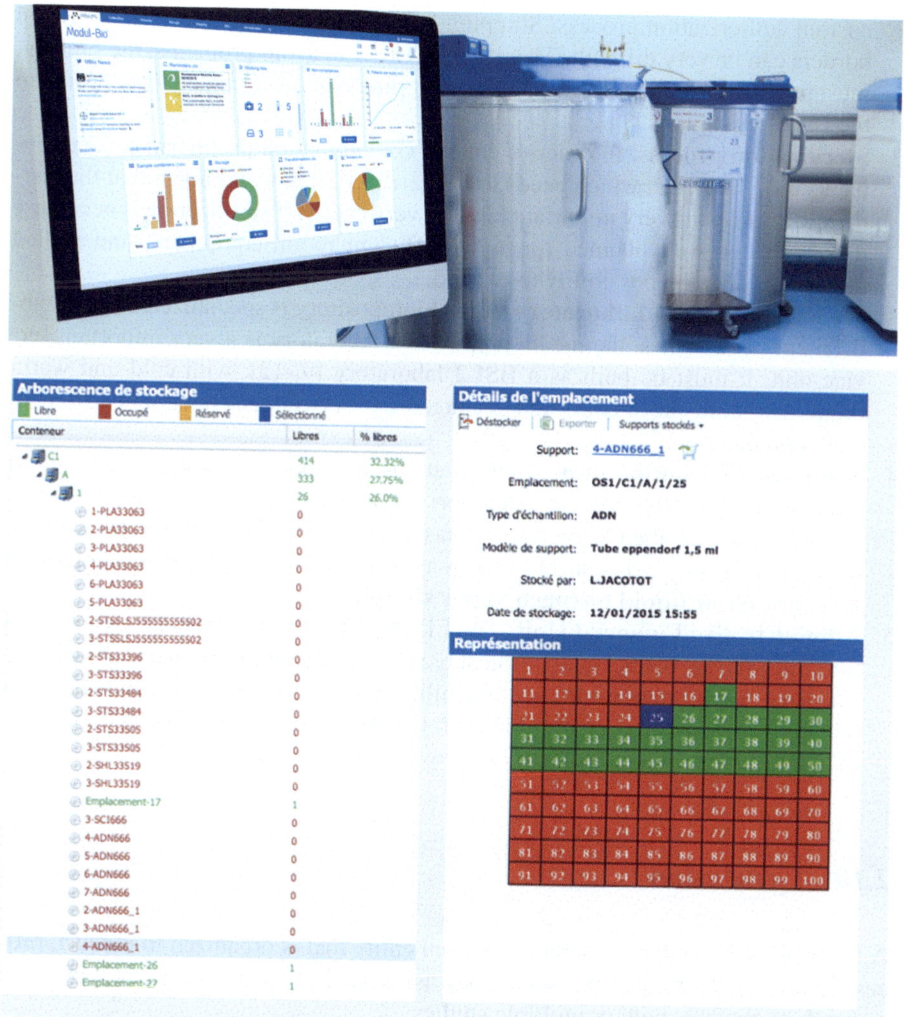

Fig. 2.13 Biobanking LIMS screen shot

specific reagents (e.g., EDTA, ACD, PaxGene, etc.) according to the type of the biological material and process (e.g., ACD for DNA extraction, PaxGene for RNA extraction, etc.); (2) a butterfly needle for standardization of blood collection; (3) Packing instruction; (4) shipping material (carton box, packing materials according to ADR or IATA regulations); and (5) preprinted shipping labels. The use of a preassembled collection kit will prevent errors during the collection of the biological material and will ensure use of the proper International Air Transport Association (IATA) shipping container, avoiding delays during the custom authorization process. Shipping biological material across international borders can be very difficult. Therefore, in order to avoid problems, the biobank must provide the collection sites with a shipping container prepared according to the IATA regulations [11].

2. **Sterilization process.** In order to control contamination problems, several biobanks use glassware, which needs to be sterilized. It is well known that the sterilization process is very important but also very costly. If sterilization is necessary it needs to be well planned for, with sufficient room, equipment, and skilled personnel, with the possibility to expand.
3. **Media preparation Laboratory**. If the biorepository is specialized in the establishment of cell lines, the media preparation laboratory is a very important service unit. It must be built as a BSL2 laboratory [9, 12], with cold and warm rooms (to store the media) and managed by skilled personnel specialized in media preparation.
4. **Shipping/Distribution unit**. After receiving the approved work order and the biomaterial from the process laboratory (which will supply not only the biospecimen but also the QC report or datasheet) the shipping unit will prepare the material to be shipped in specific IATA approved containers for **room temperature, dry ice or liquid nitrogen vapor shipping.**
5. **Administrative/Financial Unit**. The LIMS, automatically, should also send to the requester, the invoice with the cost recovery price for the biomaterial shipped. This step is important for the sustainability of the Biobank and for the ability to recover some operative costs. However, the ability to recover costs is dependent on the local institutional rules and/or government regulations.

2.10 Conclusion

A Biobank is defined as an actual or virtual entity that is organized to receive, process, store, or distribute specimens and associated clinical data in support of a research or clinical study or multiple studies.

The mission of the Biobank should address the specific purpose for which the Biobank is constituted. The mission shall be reviewed over time to ensure that it is still appropriate for the needs of the Scientific Community considering that the surrounding conditions (e.g., technological advancement; social and political environment; public health, etc.) may require a change or adaptation of the Biobank to the new needs (e.g., Covid-19 pandemic [10]).

It is important that the equipment, facilities, staffing, and funding for the Biobank be established according to a structure that will support the mission and activities during the anticipated lifecycle of the Biobank. Policies must be created, enforced, and reviewed on a regular basis concerning specimen access, handling, destruction of samples, and the potential for the termination of the Biobank.

The availability of high-quality biological and environmental specimens for research purposes requires the development of standardized methods for collection, long-term storage, retrieval, and distribution of specimens that will enable their future use. This approach requires the implementation of a Quality Management System (QMS), certified according to ISO 9001-2015 [4] standard and/or accreditation to ISO 20387:2018 [6] or College of American Pathologists (CAP) [5]).

The Biobank infrastructure needs to be designed and implemented with state-of-the-art technologies, to ensure the highest safety and operational standards and with the objective to be operative for periods up to 20–30 years and managed and operated by "structured" high skilled personnel. The commitment of the institution is critical to achieving this goal.

The technology which will be implemented (e.g., liquid nitrogen, mechanical freezers, processing equipment, etc.) must be selected to meet both present and future needs. Choices between manual and robotized equipments must be made, looking at future requirements and the possibility to improve the quality of the biospecimens. Backup systems (electrical and LN_2), remote backup, disaster plan, and sufficient space to expand are also mandatory for correct implementation and management of a Biobank.

The Process Laboratories are important to guarantee the highest quality of the biospecimen stored and distributed but must also be used to develop new procedures and standards to improve the quality of the biological material and shared with the Biobanking scientific community.

The Biobank must also be part of International Biobanking Societies and Networks (e.g., ISBER, ESBB, BBMRI, etc.) and have in the scope the goal to share the biological material collected, processed, and stored with the highest quality standard.

References

1. OECD. Best practice guidelines for biological resource centres. http://www.oecd-ilibrary.org/science-and-technology/oecd-best-practice-guidelines-for-biological-resource-centres_9789264128767-en
2. NCI best practices for biospecimen resources. http://biospecimens.cancer.gov/bestpractices/
3. ISBER. Best practice for biorepositories. http://www.isber.org/?page=BPR
4. ISO/IEC 9001:2015. Quality management systems requirements. https://www.iso.org/obp/ui/#iso:std:iso:9001:ed-5:v1:en
5. CAP Biorepository Accreditation Program. https://www.cap.org/laboratory-improvement/accreditation
6. ISO 20387:2018, Biotechnology—Biobanking—General requirements for biobanking. https://www.iso.org/standard/67888.html
7. ISBER Biobank assessment tool. https://www.isber.org/page/BAT
8. ISBER Biobank Proficiency Testing Program. https://www.isber.org/page/PTGI
9. SPIDIA self-assessment tool for molecular diagnostics to check pre-analytical workflows. https://www.spidia.eu/
10. World Health Organization (WHO). Good Laboratory Practice (GLP). https://www.who.int/tdr/publications/documents/glp-trainer.pdf

11. Centres for Disease Control and Prevention (CDC). Interim guidelines for collecting, handling, and testing clinical specimens for COVID-19. https://www.cdc.gov/coronavirus/2019-nCoV/lab/guidelines-clinical-specimens.html
12. Centres for Disease Control and Prevention (CDC) Guideline—biosafety level 2 (BSL2). Constructed according to: biosafety in Microbiological and Biomedical Laboratories. https://www.cdc.gov/labs/pdf/CDC-BiosafetyMicrobiologicalBiomedicalLaboratories-2009-P.PDF
13. ISO/TC 212. Clinical laboratory testing and in vitro diagnostic test systems. https://www.iso.org/committee/54916.html
14. BBMRI-ERIC quality management services for basic and applied research. https://www.bbmri-eric.eu/services/quality-management/
15. BBMRI-ERIC—EU General Data Protection Regulation (GDPR). http://www.bbmri-eric.eu/wp-content/uploads/BBMRI-ERIC_FAQs_on_the_GDPR_V2.0.pdf
16. Guide to shipping biological materials. http://www.ncsu.edu/ehs/dot/Bio_shipping.pdf
17. De Blasio P. and Biunno I - New Challanges for Biobanks: Accreditation to the New ISO 20387:2018 Standard Specific for Biobanks - BioTech 2021, 10,13. https://doi.org/10.3390/biotech10030013 https://doi.org/10.3390/biotech10030013

Chapter 3
Biocomputing for Biobanks: Workflow and Information Management Systems for Biobanks

Cheryl Michels

Abstract Information management systems for biobanks have grown and changed over the past 20 years. The critical need for accurate, timely, and complete information about the valuable samples stored in our biobanks continues. Without ready access to this metadata, translational medicine progress will be slowed. While a consensus exists regarding the importance of the Biobank Information Management System (BIMS), there continues to be some confusion and wariness about the size and scope of such a system. Biobank managers are undecided about what data is critical and where the data should reside. Organizations that house biobanks have conflicting priorities regarding cost containment, security, privacy, and informatics control. In the end, the dizzying array of options, programs, regulations, standards, conventions, and best practices can lead to a very unsettling approach to information management. In this chapter, we will strive to make our way through this maze and offer some practical advice on the selection, configuration, and use of a BIMS.

Keywords Biobank information management system · Information management best practices · Software for biobanks · Workflow management in biobanks

3.1 History

Back in 1986, when I started working with a laboratory at the University of Washington, there was little in the way of information management systems for small to medium-sized facilities. The personal computer had only been available for a couple of years, and computerized systems were limited to central coordinating centers and large centralized hospital systems. Cancer research probably had the most sophisticated systems for information management, but even so it meant

C. Michels (✉)
Freezerworks, a Division of Dataworks Development, Inc., Mountlake Terrace, WA, USA
e-mail: Cheryl@freezerworks.com

P. Hainaut et al. (eds.), *Biobanking of Human Biospecimens*,
https://doi.org/10.1007/978-3-030-55901-4_3

collecting data by hand on forms that were then mailed or faxed to a central location for rekeying into a mainframe computer.

In 1996, a brief analysis of the quality of hand-entered data concluded that a 20% rate of transcription error was the expected standard [1]. During the late 1980s and through the 90s, the proliferation of desktop computers began to erode the centralized control of data entry and provided researchers with the ability to collect, manage, and analyze their own data. Distributing information management was not without contention; proponents of centralized data management were concerned over the diminishment of data quality, and limited, controlled access to the data itself. Researchers and clinicians heralded the change as it meant individual control over the data they generated, supporting a sense of ownership. Of course, this ownership sometimes flew in the face of the institution's policies and the federal government's proprietary hold on the data and research. Ownership of the samples often conflicted with ownership of the data. This was particularly clear during the heady days of early AIDS research when repositories were being established all over the country: in universities, pharmaceutical companies, and government laboratories; and research was moving at a very fast pace. Whatever side of the argument you choose, it is credible that ready universal access to the data contributed in no small way to the progression of our understanding of the disease and how to combat it.

Rights to data access and access to the samples became a hot issue again after September 11, 2001. It was quickly apparent that select agents needed to be secured, and access to them and their concomitant data required control. New US federal laws were passed, Homeland Security expanded its control, and fines were assessed against those who were not properly managing their sample data [2].

On February 20, 2003, the United States Department of Health and Human Services released Health Insurance Reform, Security Standards, and the Final Rule for 45 CFR Parts 160, 162, and 164, implementing some of the requirements of the Health Insurance Portability and Accountability Act (HIPAA). This further impacted and fueled the conflict between centralized data storage and management and distributed systems that offered easy access to researchers and clinicians alike.

So, we come to today. The need and expectation for quality, secure, information management systems for biobanks is greater than ever. Organizations are looking for global solutions. Stakeholders around the world discuss, laud, and clamor for, harmonization, standardization, and interoperability. These are all good things, or at least they sound good in print, but we must not forget the human element. Individuals see the world differently. They think differently [3]. They behave differently [4]. And every biobank has its own character. Some are just banks for biological material—you deposit and you withdraw. Others invest your material in research, performing tests and reporting results. Each may require more or less functionality in a sample management information system, but there are common needs for all: data integrity, quality, traceability, ease of use. Let us explore these now.

3.2 Essential Elements of a Biobank Information Management System (BIMS)

What is an information management system for samples/biobanks? When I was working at the University of Washington in 1983, our information management system consisted of a storage closet full of logbooks. Graduate students and research assistants had, for years, painstakingly written down information about each and every sample stored in our freezers: source, type, date stored, and location. As department manager, I was tasked with the management of pulling samples for a new study on mycoplasma. Looking at the pile of logbooks, I realized that our information management system could, perhaps, be improved upon. Fast forward 30 years and what is the current state of information management systems in biobanks? Well, the Informatics Working Group of the International Society for Biological and Environmental Repositories (ISBER) conducted surveys of its members in 2010 [5] and 2012 [6]. The results were varied—respondents indicated a collection of tools were used to manage their data including paper logbooks, electronic spreadsheets, homegrown database systems, and commercial "off the shelf" software. And when viewing the landscape of commercial software, there appears a myriad of choices ranging from glorified spreadsheets to sophisticated enterprise solutions (Figs. 3.1 and 3.2).

For purposes of this discussion, we will limit our definition of a Biobank Information Management System (BIMS) to software systems built on a foundation of a relational database. While paper logbooks and electronic spreadsheets are technically speaking data management systems, they lack many of the critical features we will be discussing here.

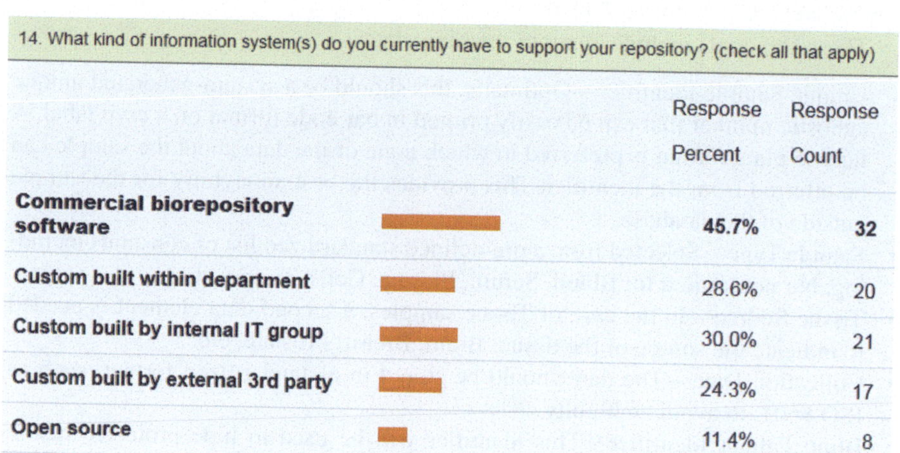
14. What kind of information system(s) do you currently have to support your repository? (check all that apply)

	Response Percent	Response Count
Commercial biorepository software	**45.7%**	**32**
Custom built within department	28.6%	20
Custom built by internal IT group	30.0%	21
Custom built by external 3rd party	24.3%	17
Open source	11.4%	8

Fig. 3.1 Results of 2010 ISBER Informatics Survey

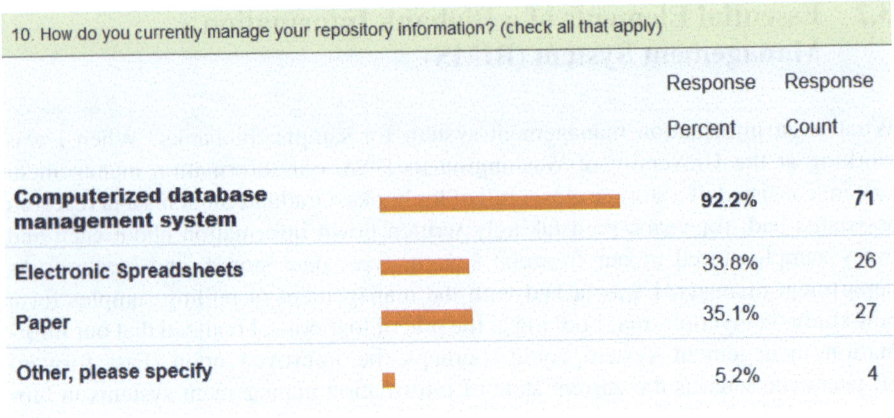

Fig. 3.2 Results of 2012 ISBER Informatics Survey

3.2.1 Minimal Dataset

There have been a number of attempts to establish a robust set of standards and best practices for the development and use of BIMS. In the United States, both ISBER [7] and the Biorepositories and Biospecimen Research Branch (BBRB) of the National Cancer Institute have published guidelines [8]. Additionally, in 2010 the Tissue Banks and Pathology Tools (TBPT) Workspace of the caBIG community defined the Common Biorepository Module (CBM) which detailed the content and format for a minimal dataset [9]. The ESBBperanto Working Group of the European, Middle Eastern, and African Society for Biopreservation and Biobanking (ESBB) was formed in 2011 to "enable comparability of biomaterials and data across different biobanks and countries." [10].

These standards include many of the same data:

- Unique Sample Identifier—Optimally, this should be a system-generated unique agnostic number that can be easily printed in bar code format on a cryo label. A license plate format is preferred in which none of the data about the sample can be inferred from the identifier. This provides the best anonymity for the sample outside of the database.
- Sample Type—Selected from a pre-defined standardized list of constants including, but not limited to: Blood, Serum, Plasma, Cells, Tissue, etc.
- Tissue Source—In the case of Tissue samples, a second data element is needed to indicate the source of the tissue: Brain, Breast, Prostate, etc.
- Collection Date—The date should be stored in a standardized format, such as ISO 8601, to avoid ambiguity.
- Blind Patient Identifier—This identifier will be used to hide protected health information when appropriate while providing the honest broker with a means to find specific patient samples if necessary.

To put it simply, a BIMS must be able to clearly and unambiguously identify a sample, its source, and relevant metadata, all the while protecting the privacy of the human being from whence it came. However, if important, potentially life-altering, results are obtained from a given sample, there must also be a way to return those results to the patient.

3.2.2 *Workflow Management*

Storing essential data about the samples in the biobank is only one element of a quality BIMS. Biobanks have numerous jobs to do and the BIMS must support that system. Because the range of tasks performed by biobanks varies, the following may or may not be essential to any given implementation of a BIMS:

- Planning and Scheduling.
- Sample Collection.
- Sample Accession.
- Sample Processing.
- Storage.
- Retrieval.
- Shipping.
- Testing.
- Billing.

3.2.2.1 Planning and Scheduling

Finite resources (money, supplies, manpower) dictate that a biobank manager be able to anticipate the number of samples to be received, processed, stored, and shipped during a given time period. A valuable workflow management tool in a BIMS includes the ability to set up pre-defined clinical trials project plans, which will be used to store that information, modify it as realities change, and generate useful reports of anticipated needed resources.

3.2.2.2 Sample Collection

Some biobanks collect data about the patient/donor and the sample itself at the time the sample is drawn. Mobile devices can be especially useful at this point, becoming more common in many clinical settings. Electronic laboratory notebooks (ELN) have already been used for a number of years to collect this data. Storing the data electronically at the point of collection reduces the possibility of transcription error and improves the general quality of the data. In the case where the biobank is closely allied to the clinic, this becomes the first step in the electronic chain of data management. Assigning a unique identifier to each sample obtained is critical to this chain.

3.2.2.3 Sample Accession

Many biobanks receive samples after collection without having any control or participation in that process. In some cases, samples arrive with printed forms containing critical data. In others, tubes arrive with a combination of handwritten/computer-generated labels. In both of these cases, the biobank must transcribe the data into the BIMS. To reduce transcription error, the BIMS ideally will have built-in, yet configurable, data integrity checks. These may include, but are not limited to, domain checking (e.g., sample types from an approved dropdown list), range checking (e.g., dates must be within a sensible, configured range), and referential integrity (e.g., gender dictates allowable sample types).

Configurable business rules that populate data automatically will also reduce transcription error and improve efficiency. Simple examples include automatically setting the Collection Date to yesterday or Date Received to today. Slightly more complex examples include populating a set of common protocol-related data elements based on the protocol selected (e.g., Protocol ABC enrolls only females, so Gender is automatically populated accordingly). The user should always be able to override these default values, should an exception need to be made (e.g., while most samples are entered into the database on the day they are received, there could be exceptions to that).

If the samples arrive at the biobank without a unique identifier, the BIMS must assign one at the point of accession to begin the electronic chain.

3.2.2.4 Sample Processing

Steps taken in processing the sample are critical to maintaining its quality, and, therefore, the quality of the data generated by it downstream. The Biospecimen Working Group of ISBER identified critical pre-analytical factors for biospecimen sample processing and developed a Standard Preanalytical Code (SPREC) to record these data points in a coded fashion [11]. It is important for the BIMS to store these data in order to provide assurances to future researchers of the quality of the samples. While SPREC is one way to code this data in a standardized fashion, it is not essential to use it. Data about the processing of the specimen can be discretely stored in the BIMS in a manner that makes retrieval and analysis possible. And, should the science of biospecimen processing change such that critical values like centrifugation speeds/times change, the use of discrete data points in the BIMS will have the advantage over coded systems that pre-define these data points without any option to change. The more raw data stored the better chance of quality analysis in the future.

3.2.2.5 Storage

It seems simplistic to say, but it does no good to store samples in a biobank if they cannot be found when needed. No one would place their property in public storage without the locker number and a key to the front gate. Critical data in the BIMS include the storage date, volume/quantity stored, and exact storage location. Data integrity checks at this point include preventing two samples from being stored in the same freezer position. In some cases, the freezer store selection is based on configurable elements such as sample type (e.g., cells are stored in LN2 while serum is stored in mechanical freezers). Business rules that allow users to default the volume or quantity stored based on the sample type can also improve the quality of the data while reducing keyboard time.

3.2.2.6 Retrieval

As above, if samples cannot be retrieved accurately, the biobank has failed its primary mission. Users must be able to search the BIMS by any piece of data stored and retrieve a list of matching samples and their exact freezer locations. Automated stores make this function less error prone and provide protected, temperature-controlled access to the desired samples. Once the desired samples have been identified and located, the BIMS should provide an easy way to check them out of the system, either temporarily or permanently, clearing the freezer position or holding it for return of the samples. Additional data elements to be saved at this step may include the date of the removal, the name of the person who removed the samples, an increment to the number of thaws, and the eventual disposition of the samples.

3.2.2.7 Shipping

Once samples have been retrieved from storage, they may need to be shipped to another facility. The BIMS should provide tools to create a shipping manifest (printed and electronic), store information about the eventual destination of the shipment, and track the shipment using the shipper's tracking identifier. All information about the shipment should be searchable in the future so that at any time the biobank manager can determine in which shipment an individual sample was included.

3.2.2.8 Testing

Some, but certainly not all, biobanks perform testing on samples based on the requirements of the specific clinical trial. For those biobanks, it is critical that the BIMS provides tools to order tests, import results, and generate results reports. In these cases, protecting patient identity may be even more critical (more on that later). In some biobanks, a secondary software program actually manages the testing data, and the BIMS needs to integrate with it so that results can be linked back to the stored samples and vice versa.

3.2.2.9 Billing

Finally, for some biobanks, the business of banking is revenue generating. In these situations, having an integrated billing module in the BIMS is important. The system should, at minimum, allow the biobank to generate invoices or billing data for repository services provided by day, month, or year, according to the individual contract. In most cases, there will be different charge rates for different types of samples due to the varying costs of LN2, vapor phase, and mechanical freezers. Biobanks may also charge for services such as DNA extraction, cell line growth, or resuscitation of oocytes. And, if tests are performed within the biobank, they may need to charge for those as well.

3.2.2.10 Workflow in Summary

Workflow management in a BIMS should incorporate all of the tasks performed in a biobank, allowing for varying entry points in the process, and providing integration with other systems when necessary. The primary objectives are to (1) eliminate transcription error at all points; (2) provide the best quality of data to the final recipient of the sample; and (3) alleviate the effort required by the biobank staff to store and retrieve samples and their data.

3.2.3 Security, Privacy, and Other Regulatory Issues

Regulatory issues covering security and privacy have continued to grow in importance on the international stage. While a BIMS cannot itself be compliant with regulations, it must provide all of the tools so that its users can comply with those regulations that are applicable. This includes, but is not limited to, a user/password system, controlled permissions/roles for various functions within the software, the ability to hide specified data from unauthorized users, the ability to track automatically any and all changes to the data, and finally the ability to track all views of Personal Health Information (PHI).

3.2.3.1 System Security

The BIMS must include a mechanism to authenticate users of the system, either separately or in conjunction with the domain server using the Lightweight Directory Access Protocol (LDAP). Different organizations will have different user name and password requirements and the BIMS should be flexible enough to allow the most restrictive rules to be enforced without requiring them for those biobanks where security is less critical.

Most biobanks will want to prevent unauthorized users from performing specific functions within the software through the definition of roles (e.g., Accession, Storage and Retrieval, Shipping, Search Only, etc.). These functions may differ from biobank to biobank and should therefore be configurable by the user rather than pre-defined.

In addition to prevent unauthorized functions, many biobanks have the concept of sample ownership. Customers of the biobank may require access to their sample data without the ability to see other customers' data. Therefore, the BIMS must provide record-level access configuration so that biobanks can hide one customer's sample data from other customers.

Finally, only honest brokers, or their designees, should ever have access to PHI. While this may be set up as a Role above, it crosses the workflow functions and requires the protection of individual pieces of data. Therefore, it should be handled separately.

3.2.3.2 Audit Trail

The ISBER Best Practices document states that the Audit trail must be an automatic, non-editable, record of all changes made to the data in the BIMS [7]. At minimum, it must include the name of the user making the change, the date and time of the change, the data element name, both the original value and the new value, and, in some cases, the reason for the change [12]. When storing the date and time of the change, it is critical to use a common time zone in those cases where users of the BIMS are in disparate geographical locations. Use of the ISO 8601 date standard is an easy solution [13]. The Audit Trail should be searchable, but not editable. It must provide an accurate and convenient method to find all changes made to data stored on a given sample. In addition, it should allow an easy way to find all changes made to data by a given individual, in the case of a question about the quality of the data entry of that individual. And, the Audit Trail should also provide a history of a given freezer location, showing all samples ever stored in the location by date and time (in the case of a reported system store issue).

3.2.3.3 Record of Viewing of PHI

HIPAA requires that biobanks, and others, be able to provide to any individual a list of names and dates of anyone who viewed their PHI. See 45 C.F.R. § 164.528. The BIMS should include an automated record of all viewing of PHI by user name, date, time, and what PHI was viewed. "Viewing" includes any and all potential access to the PHI including report generation and external access to the data.

3.3 Gaining Compliance: How Do We Get People to Use the System?

There is an old saying about horses and water that applies to any software program, and the BIMS is no exception. Given how much benefit is gained from the proper use of a BIMS, why would it not be embraced fully? What are the obstacles to full implementation? And how can we overcome these obstacles to improve the quality of work-life and data in the biobank?

3.3.1 Legacy Systems

One of the first obstacles encountered by any biobank in its efforts to establish and implement a new BIMS is the legacy system. New biobanks, of course, do not have this challenge, but, existing collections often have 1000s of samples stored in freezers throughout the organization in a myriad of box sizes and storage systems. The data associated with those samples may even be in logbooks, electronic spreadsheets, and homegrown databases that no one knows how to access, or in no longer supported commercial systems. Unfortunately, the quality of the data may be compromised. The monumental task of verifying the inventory against the data stored in the legacy system may be so onerous that no one wants to even begin. Breaking through the status quo to establish a system even with the legacy still in place is required. It is better to get new samples stored and cataloged correctly sooner rather than later. (The migration of data from legacy systems into a new BIMS will be discussed later.) There are organizations that will contract with biobanks to perform a physical inventory of legacy samples and clean up the data to match what is in the inventory. As crazy as it sounds, there is also a school of thought that suggests that if the quality of the data is compromised, it may not be worth the effort to salvage the legacy samples. In these times of limited resources, should biobanks be using energy to store samples that may never be used because we simply do not know what we have? [14].

3.3.2 Resistance to Change

Regardless of the numerous excellent features included in a BIMS, if the end users do not embrace it, it will likely sit on a shelf gathering dust. And, no matter how challenging or error prone the current system/methodology for tracking repository data, there is frequently a resistance to change. This is human nature and volumes have been written about change management in the past 50 years. Adopting some of the basic tenets of change management and applying them to the implementation process for a new BIMS will increase the chances of success. The first step is to get all of the end users of the system, both current and potential, to identify the challenges with the current system. Most people are willing to talk about what is not working well for them, even if they do not want to change. If the end users are candid, this exercise will generate a starting point for the features needed in any new BIMS—features that are meaningful to the current users. For example, if the current system uses electronic spreadsheets to store the data, the challenges may include an inability to search across all the spreadsheets for a discrete set of samples that meet needed criteria. Or, the level of effort necessary to annotate each sample may be quite high. Of course, the most serious challenge with electronic spreadsheets is the lack of data integrity checking, which can result in less than high-quality data.

Next, the end users should be asked to identify those features of their current system that they simply cannot live without. Using the example of the spreadsheets again, these may include ease of use (everyone is familiar with spreadsheets), ability to change the columns at will without engaging a professional software developer, and a feeling of ownership ("I created this spreadsheet to meet my very specific needs").

3.3.3 Why Do So Many Global, Enterprise Solutions Fail?

The biobank informatics landscape is littered with global/enterprise solutions that sounded good in print but failed in action. Millions of dollars have been spent developing these solutions, all for naught [15]. While no scientific study has been conducted to determine the causes of these failures, we may be permitted to make some educated guesses based on intuition and experience.

1. One size does not fit all. Global enterprise solutions focus, understandably, on standardization. Everyone must do everything in the same way. This sounds like a laudable goal. How can we possibly share data, maximize efficiency, and gain economies of scale if everyone is doing their own thing? The problem is that too often the lowest common denominator satisfies no one, and therefore no one uses it. Or, at the other extreme, the global solution includes everything that all stakeholders require, resulting in a system so complex and confusing that no one can use it.

2. Stakeholders have competing, and sometimes mutually exclusive, requirements. This is evident in both the private sector and the public sector. Often, the global IT professional is looking for an integrated, familiar solution that meets a list of preset requirements designed to ease their incredibly challenging responsibilities of ensuring quality and security across the organization. At the other end of the global spectrum sits the end user in the biobank whose most critical need is a system that is easy to use, accessible, and mitigates their incredibly challenging responsibility of managing the day-to-day tasks of the high throughput biobank. Finding a solution that meets both sets of needs frequently comes down to who has the most power in the organization. When the expressed immediate needs of the end users are set aside in order to meet the perceived global needs of the organization, what often results is a lack of compliance on the part of the end users.
3. Managers of standardized enterprise solutions are frequently unable to respond to the changing needs and requirements of the end users. Since the BIMS is standardized for the entire organization, change requests often have to be vetted by a corporate oversight group. These requests then are put into a queue and prioritized against all other requests from the organization. A critical change for one biobank in an organization may be irrelevant to most other users. A good example of this is the need to track a new piece of data for a small pilot research program—because no one else needs to track this data, its priority in the organization as a whole is low. The result is the biobank may begin to use electronic spreadsheets to track the data outside the BIMS. After a few of these types of requests, the biobank may simply decide that it is easier to use their own homegrown system rather than the enterprise solution, or, they maintain a shadow system and enter all of the data twice.

3.3.4 So, How Do We Improve Compliance?

A BIMS that balances standardization and configurability provides the best of both worlds.

- Define a minimal dataset ensuring that each user of the BIMS collects the data required by the enterprise.
- Allow each business unit to define specific data elements that are in addition to this minimal dataset.
- Define established workflow protocols for those procedures that must be identical across the organization.
- Allow each business unit to define additional workflows in the BIMS to meet their unique and idiosyncratic requirements.
- Allow trained representatives from each business unit to make configuration changes to the BIMS that are within their scope.

The key here is to ensure that the overall needs of the organization are met while the individual needs of the business units are fully addressed. In this way, compliance with the use of the BIMS will be less of a struggle.

3.4 Build Versus Buy

A question that comes up frequently and that many organizations struggle with is whether to purchase a commercial "off the shelf" software program for their BIMS, to build one from scratch, or to create a hybrid of some sort. There is no one right answer, but there are pros and cons for each. The 2012 ISBER Informatics Working Group Survey summarized the types of systems that were in use by the respondents [6] (Fig. 3.3).

3.4.1 Building a System

Using your own resources to building a system from scratch increases the chance that your system will meet your exact workflow needs. In addition, you will only get the features that you actually need, with no extraneous complexity. Intimate involvement in the process of development can produce high-quality results. That quality can come at a price. Development time and costs can be quite high because everything must be built from scratch. A bigger problem is the potential lack of

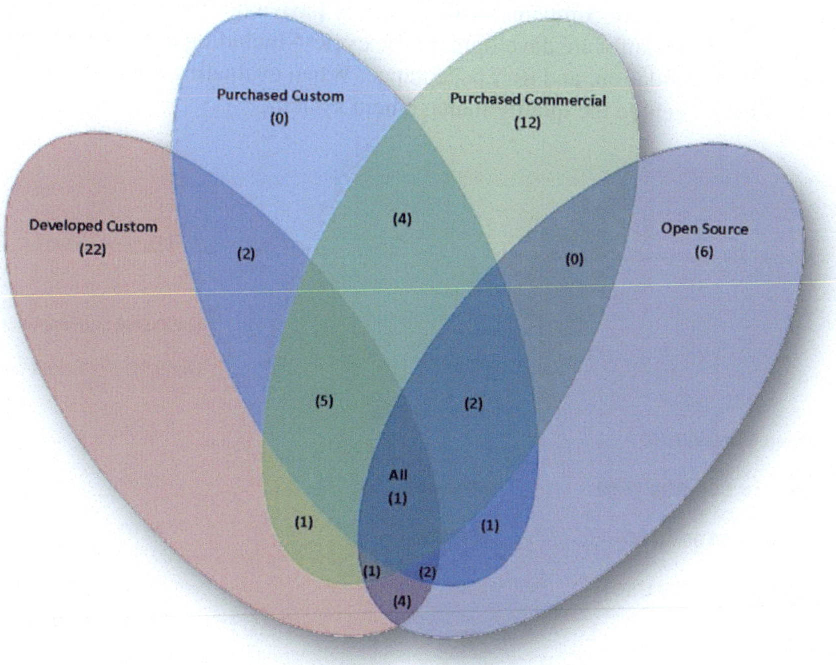

Fig. 3.3 Breakdown of Systems Used in Biobanks—2012 Informatics Survey

sustainability. If the original development team leaves the organization, it can be very difficult to provide continuous support.

If you are building your own system, you also need to ensure that you have the quality assurance programs in place to govern the software development life cycle. Documentation at every stage is critical in order to ensure the continued value of the system. Validation of the software must be completed and must include both the software development lifecycle as well as the use of the system and validation of the user requirements.

3.4.2 *Purchasing a Commercial off-the-Shelf Program*

Commercial, off-the-shelf, software programs vary widely in cost and features. As an example, the 2012 ISBER Informatics Survey reported the following (Fig. 3.4):

This is a small sample but is likely indicative of the range in costs.

Many of the implementation details required in a biobank have already been addressed, often reducing the time to program initiation. Since these systems are built for a large number of customers, there may be features that you do not need, adding to the cost of purchasing and learning the system. Conversely, there may be desirable features that are excluded.

Commercial software companies will generally have a quality management system that governs the software development life cycle—including user requirements, design, coding, validation, and user acceptance. When evaluating commercial software, be sure to include the quality management system.

28. What was the approximate initial cost (in USD) of the software, including any required implementation or installation costs?

	Response Percent	Response Count
Less than $10,000 USD	0.0%	0
$10,000 to $50,000 USD	**32.0%**	**8**
$50,000 to $100,000 USD	28.0%	7
$100,000 to $250,000 USD	16.0%	4
$250,000 to $500,000 USD	12.0%	3
More than $500,000 USD	12.0%	3

Fig. 3.4 2012 ISBER Informatics Survey

Ongoing support and training are critical to maintaining the value of your investment. With that in mind, carefully evaluate the availability and the quality of the support and training offered by the commercial software company.

3.4.3 Using Open Source Code to Develop a System

The use of "free" open source code has waxed and waned over the past 10 years. The mantra of many finance-conscious individuals has been "free is good." It is important to remember another old saying, "you get what you pay for," or one of my father's favorites, "there are no free lunches." While open source code is often available for no initial cash outlay, it has been suggested by the National Cancer Institute's OBBR that the cost to implement such an open source solution in a biobank is close to the cost for one of the larger enterprise commercial software solutions [16]. A programmer must learn the style of the individual who wrote the open source code and understand his design decisions before he can modify or enhance it. This can take months of hard work, depending upon the level of documentation and adherence to standards. Open source code may or may not adhere to a standard, or it may not be evident what standard is being used. Furthermore, the design decisions made by the original developer can dictate how enhancements must be done, or limit the possibilities.

3.5 How to Choose a BIMS

There are a number of steps and criteria that will increase your chances of building or purchasing the right system for your organization:

- Identify essential workflows and processes.
- Define and prioritize user requirements.
- Evaluate quality management systems.
- Time for implementation.
- Cost of implementation.
- Cost of ownership.

3.5.1 Identify Essential Workflows and Processes

What processes or workflows are followed in your biobank? As you identify these, keep in mind those workflows that were created because of a limitation in your existing information management system. For example, some biobanks use electronic spreadsheets to track accessioning of samples because their existing system does not generate a unique identifier for each sample received. This process, while essential with the existing system, should be unnecessary with a new or updated BIMS.

3.5.2 Define and Prioritize User Requirements

Based on the workflows identified, define a list of all user requirements. Be sure to include all stakeholders in the development of this list: from the IT professional to the accessioning desk to the honest broker to the financial director to the shipping clerk. Collecting and balancing the requirements of all potential users of the system is critical in the early stage to increase compliance and user acceptance. Carefully listen to end users as much as possible—their day-to-day use of the system is the end result of your investment.

Once all of the requirements have been listed, prioritize them. This can be as simple as having each stakeholder assign a numeric value to each. This prioritized list can then be used to compare the various options available in a systematic way.

3.5.3 Evaluate Quality Management Systems

The long-term quality of the software selected or built can be to some extent extrapolated from the quality of the management system used to develop and support it. When purchasing a commercial software program, look carefully at the quality management system (QMS) of the company. Ask to see documentation of the QMS and of the validation performed on the software. When selecting an open source solution or building your own from scratch, perform the same evaluation of the internal QMS.

Because the biobank is storing patient samples, the BIMS may store sensitive patient information. Thus, compliance with ever increasing regulations governing this information may depend, in part, on the QMS.

3.5.4 Time for Implementation

They say that "time is money." How critical is timely implementation? Sometimes, the onset of a new study or the expected receipt of a large number of samples can dictate a speedy implementation.

The ISBER Informatics Survey [6] collected information on the time required for implementation, comparing the various options. There was no clear pattern available, with time ranging from weeks to years. If you are evaluating commercial software, ask the vendor to provide a written timeline for implementation and user acceptance. If building your own, you need to develop a similar project plan. Use of commercial project planning software can aid in tracking whether the project is on time and on budget.

3.5.5 *Cost of Implementation*

When purchasing a commercial package, ask the vendor to clearly identify what is and is not included in the stated price: licensing fees, number of users (simultaneous or named), installation, training, implementation, support (how much and for how long), or upgrades. Make sure to add in any labor costs for biobank staff to learn and validate the software.

When building a system, determine the number of hours and associated costs of each staff member involved, including software developers, validators, trainers, and support staff. This is important but sometimes overlooked, as the cost of biobank staff is fixed. However, if biobank staff members are spending 20 h per week evaluating iterative versions of the built software, they are not spending those hours performing the business of the biobank, and that is a cost that must be enumerated.

Finally, determine the cost to migrate any existing data into the new system (see below for a discussion of this important step).

3.5.6 *Cost of Ownership*

This was included above but is worthy of a second mention. When comparing the options, be sure to clarify the cost to support the system for its expected lifetime (e.g., 5, 10, and 20 years). Additionally, estimate the cost of upgrading the system to accommodate new hardware such as computers, labeling systems, automated cryo-stores, mobile technology, etc., as well as the changing landscape of biobanking with new standards, guidelines, and accreditation requirements. Is the system capable of agile adaptation to these changes and how costly will the changes be?

3.5.7 *Making the Choice*

Once you have answered all of the questions, evaluated all of the options, and narrowed down the choices, you have to pick one. Because there is no one right decision, there is a bit of educated guessing to do. If you are leaning towards a commercial software package, you can decrease your guessing and increase your assurance by talking with other users of the preferred package. Find out what they like and do not like about the software and the company providing it. If you are leaning towards building your own system, with or without open source code, talk to other organizations that have done the same. Learn from their experiences to increase your own chance of success.

3.6 Data Migration

Once you have selected a solution for your BIMS, you may have legacy data that needs to be migrated into the new system. This legacy data may be in handwritten logbooks, electronic spreadsheets, flat file databases, homegrown systems, or archaic customized systems. Common to all of these sources of data are the following questions or issues:

- Data Quality—What is the general quality of the data? Depending on the existence and type of data integrity checking done in the existing system, the data may require a lot of "cleaning" in order to be utilized and trusted. Simple data integrity includes the validity of dates, times, and expected numeric values. More complex data integrity checking may include checking for duplicates of values that are expected to be unique.
- Data Content—Are there differences in the way that the same data elements have been entered? For example, are serum sample types annotated as serum, sera, ser, s, or something else entirely? In these cases, a mapping system will need to be created to ensure that all common data elements are written to the new system in a standardized fashion.
- Storage Locations—Is there inconsistency in the way in which freezer storage locations are recorded? Are discrete locations always recorded or are some of the locations simply the box or container in which the samples are stored? This critical data can often be the most difficult to sort out during the data migration process.
- Unique Identifiers—One sometimes overlooked issue when migrating data from a variety of electronic sources is a potential overlap of unique identifiers. In those cases where more than one electronic source has been used to store the legacy data, there may be duplicates of expected unique identifiers. If these identifiers have been included on the label of the sample in storage, it is necessary to maintain the identifier in the new system, along with its source. No one wants to relabel frozen samples!
- Audit Trail—If the data is being migrated from another electronic source that contained an audit trail, a decision whether to migrate the audit trail or keep it accessible in the old system must be made. Depending on the specific requirements of your biobank, either of these solutions is possible. Most regulations allow for the audit trail to be maintained in the old system as long as it remains accessible. Alternatively, if the old system allows for a printout of the audit trail, then permanent storage of an unalterable printout will satisfy most regulatory agencies. If it is necessary to migrate the audit trail along with the data itself,

then care must be taken to ensure that the content of the audit trail is not changed during the migration and remains non-editable.

Of course, all data migrations require rigorous validation to ensure that no data is modified. This validation should include, at minimum, a check of the total count of records transferred from the old system to the new and verification of the consistency of the data on a random sampling of records between the old and the new.

3.7 Conclusion

Much is written and discussed about the importance of biobanking to the future of translational research and personalized medicine. Millions of dollars are spent each year on personnel, processing supplies, cryotubes, labels, automated stores, mechanical freezers, electricity, liquid nitrogen, etc., to process and store the veritable goldmine that constitutes our biobanks. Sadly, software has become an undervalued commodity in our high technology culture, where apps are available on smartphones at little or no cost. However, without high-quality informatics systems to manage the data associated with our valuable samples, the value of those samples decreases. It is imperative that we continue to maintain and improve our informatics systems to ensure that they support the vital work being done by and with the biobank community.

References

1. Michels C, LE (1996) Benefits of a complete laboratory management software system in HIV clinical trials. Eleventh international AIDS conference. Vancouver, BC
2. Regulations—Select Agents Regulations. (2013). Retrieved from National Select Agent Registry: http://www.selectagents.gov/Regulations.html
3. Products and Services (2014) Retrieved from Herrmann International: http://www.hbdi.com/WholeBrainProductsAndServices/programs/thehbdi.php
4. discprofile (2014) Retrieved from DiSC overview: https://www.discprofile.com/what-is-disc/overview/
5. Group I. I (2011) 2011 ISBER informatics survey. Retrieved from http://www.zoomerang.com/Shared/SharedResultsPasswordPage.aspx?ID=L24JB7Y3KAQ8
6. ISBER Informatics Working Group (2013) Best practices for choosing and implementing information systems. In: ISBER 2013 annual meeting. Sydney
7. International Society for Biological and Environmental Repositories (2012) 2012 best practices for repositories, collection, storage, retrieval, and distribution of biological materials for research
8. National Cancer Institute, National Institutes of Health, U.S. Department of Health and Human Services (2007) National Cancer Institute best practices for biospecimen resources
9. National Cancer Institute (2010) Tissue banks & pathology tools workspace. Retrieved from caBIG Community: https://wiki.nci.nih.gov/display/TBPT/Common+Biorepository+Model+%28CBM%29

10. ESBB (2012) ESBB working group on metadata: “ESBBperanto” manifesto. Retrieved from ESBB: http://www.esbb.org/download/ESBBperanto_manifesto.pdf
11. ISBER Biospecimen Science Working Group (2012) Standard preanalytical coding for biospecimens: review and implementation of the sample PREanalytical code. Biopreserv Biobank 10:366–374
12. U.S. Food and Drug Administration (2014) *FDA*. Retrieved from Part 11, Electronic Records; Electronic Signatures—Scope and Application: http://www.fda.gov/regulatoryinformation/guidances/ucm125067.htm
13. ISO (2014) Date and time format—ISO 8601. Retrieved from ISO: http://www.iso.org/iso/home/standards/iso8601.htm
14. Vaught J, RJ (2011) An NCI perspective on creating sustainable biospecimen resources. J Natl Cancer Inst Monogr 2011(42):1–7
15. Board of Scientific Advisors Ad Hoc Working Group (2011) An assessment of the impact of the NCI cancer biomedical informatics grid
16. TC (2008) The ROI case for catissue total cost of ownership. caBIG 2008 annual meeting. Washington

Chapter 4
Tissue Preservation and Factors Affecting Tissue Quality

Peter H. J. Riegman

Abstract Acquisition of reliable and reproducible results from tissue samples can be complicated due to the introduced variations in the signals to be measured during the sample pre-analytical phase. Such variations are introduced during tissue processing because the cells in the tissue are still alive and respond to their surroundings until they are conserved for future use. In addition, tissue fixation methods can even alter the chemical structure of the signals. Standardization of the pre-analytical or pre-examination processes according to ISO Technical Standards that describe the specifications for pre-examination processes can largely avoid the introduction of different incomparable variations. Since, not all steps can be standardized, the technical standards ask for documentation of these steps. This documentation can be used as sample metadata to determine if samples are fit for purpose and comparable. Highlights on how to approach and implement such standards in a biobank is discussed in more detail in this chapter.

Keywords Frozen tissue · Tissue bank · Snap freezing · Tissue sample quality · Frozen tissue QA and QC

4.1 Introduction

Tissue sample quality is crucial not only when tissues are used for diagnostics development but also for medical research. Therefore, this is one of the major leading issues for biobanking guidelines and best practices [1–5] and it will also form the backbone for evaluating how and where to freeze tissue samples, as discussed in this chapter. Frozen tissue samples are known for their high quality and the best choice for sensitive research experiments. The choice of the frozen tissue resource (surgical specimen, biopsy, or post mortem) can have quality implications. Other preservation choices like formalin-fixed and paraffin-embedded (FFPE) tissues can be of generally of low quality, but might turn out to be fit for the intended purpose and more

P. H. J. Riegman (✉)
Pathology Department, Erasmus Medical Center, Rotterdam, The Netherlands
e-mail: p.riegman@erasmusmc.nl

P. Hainaut et al. (eds.), *Biobanking of Human Biospecimens*,
https://doi.org/10.1007/978-3-030-55901-4_4

readily available than frozen tissue samples. Quality issues for frozen tissue concerning the tissue resource, collection environment, and preservation methods in practice are discussed in order to describe those aspects that can be taken into account for a tissue bank to employ a sample processing method that can deliver the high quality and fit for purpose samples needed for medical research projects. This chapter also provides information related to tissue sample quality to make the right choices in the cohort selection for tissue research projects that could serve as the basis for guidance from the biobank manager to the research team requesting tissue samples.

4.1.1 Tissue Preservation Methods Result in Different Sample Qualities

Tissues in combination with the appropriate data form a powerful source of information on disease status and disease progression when used in the appropriate way. Since the discovery of the microscope, pathologists have been able to develop diagnostic correlations on the basis of histology. Later, pathologists could further improve these skills through the addition of special stains using histochemistry and more recently immunohistochemistry. In this manner, the pathology departments were developed into centers within the hospital, where other disciplines would submit tissues (surgical specimens and biopsies) for further diagnosis. The latest important developing discipline is molecular diagnostics, where molecular techniques are used to define characteristics correlated to disease status and progression. However, revolutionary the molecular diagnostics may be, the relation with underlying histology remains a very strong and mandatory combination. Since FFPE is the sample of choice for histology, because of the best microscopic morphologic quality, molecular diagnostics preferably uses this sample type because it is readily available and well documented. Nowadays the pathology departments can best function as central facilities where the tissues are collected, processed, and documented for diagnosis, and are approached by investigators for tissues to be used for medical research.

The basis for the majority of diagnostic techniques is the FFPE tissue fragments, routinely produced and archived for the microscopic pathology examinations. They are derived from surgical specimens, biopsies, and autopsies. This archive, which forms part of the documentation of the diagnosis, can under certain conditions also be used for medical research purposes. Although FFPE can be used for many techniques, the quality of the samples and their derivatives such as DNA, RNA, or proteins are often not high enough and appropriate as fit for purpose to be used as input for very sensitive medical research analyses. The formalin fixation can even introduce chemical changes in DNA, RNA, and proteins. Freezing tissues provide samples with a higher more native quality, and for this reason many academic hospital pathology departments have dedicated medical research tissue banks containing fresh frozen tissue. The best and major source for the collection are the surgical specimens send to pathology for diagnostic purposes. Other sources for frozen tissue in the pathology setting are needle biopsies and post mortem materials.

4.2 Variations in Sample Quality

It is important to realize that variations introduced during the collection process can influence the end results of an experiment or test. The way and the magnitude in which the results are influenced depend on the test sensitivity and the effect of the variation that was introduced.

Ideally, all samples should be treated exactly the same until the moment they are used for analyses. To minimize variations during this pre-analytical phase, and assure that the collection procedures are performed in a similar way for every sample, the procedures must be described in standard operating procedures (SOPs). In addition, a competent quality assurance and quality control (QA and QC) program is needed in the biobank to check SOP compliance in terms of quality. The period before the analytical phase is referred to as the pre-analytical phase. For tissue banks the pre-analytical phase can be divided into three distinct phases: (1) the pre-acquisition phase, (2) the acquisition phase, and (3) the post-acquisition phase. See Fig. 4.1 where these phases are shown in parallel to a timeline covering specific subsequent steps in a sample life cycle.

4.2.1 *Pre-acquisition Phase*

This phase covers the period before the sample is received in the biobank and comes under the control of biobanking SOPs. In a hospital setting, this period includes the treatment of the patient in terms of medical care. Aspects differing from one patient to another such as variations of drug intake, differing surgical procedures and duration, or anesthesia can exert influences on gene expression that can differ in different organs and cell types. The time periods of warm and cold (<body temperature) ischemia (transport) can vary between the different patients and can also influence expression or cause the degradation of derivatives. Also, the general condition of the patient's genetic background and treatment of concomitant disease can play a role. These aspects cannot be controlled with standardization and will contribute to variations in sample quality.

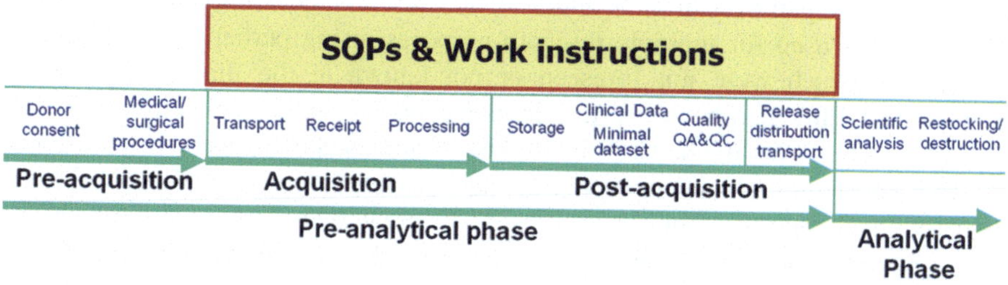

Fig. 4.1 Distinguished phases important for quality during the lifetime of a sample and where biobank SOP's and work instructions have their influence

4.2.2 Acquisition Phase

This is where the sample is transported, received in the biobank, and processed for long-term conservation and storage. This is also the start of the processes coming under control of the biobank SOPs and work instructions executed by dedicated biobank personnel. From this moment standardization can minimize the variations introduced to the sample.

4.2.3 Post-acquisition Phase

The post-acquisition phase includes the long-term storage of the sample, where further data acquisition takes place. The data collected during the earlier phases is usually about the sample characteristics, but during storage the minimal amount of information agreed to by the project leadership, including clinical data and follow-up data, are collected and stored in a dataset. This minimal dataset can be used for cohort selection and expanded at the time the samples are retrospectively used for a specific study. Prospective studies usually require another minimal dataset that can be collected during storage. In practice, the clinical departments collect the study data on their patients and use this data in combination with the minimal dataset of the samples. This model seems fragmented, but on the other hand stimulates multi-disciplinary study participation, which is better for the resulting study design and analysis. Another activity in this period is executing the QA and QC program on the collected samples.

4.3 High Quality and Fit for Purpose Samples

For research purposes, it is important to acquire samples that are fit for purpose of the tests they will be used for. This means there are quality margins where the samples do not always need to be of the highest quality. However, during the time samples are collected, which can take many years, research techniques and insights might have changed over time. In addition, new research questions can require that one sample is used for multiple research purposes, using perhaps more sensitive techniques, which were not foreseen or not known at the time of collection. Moreover, quality compatibility throughout a larger sample collection warrants flexibility in applying the latest insights. Tissues are used to answer many different research questions and serve as input material for a large array of methods and techniques with a large variety of sensitivities. These are good reasons to aim for a high-quality sample that is fit for purpose and can be used for a wide variety of analyses.

A big hurdle in minimizing variations introduced to the tissue sample during the pre-analytical phase is the pre-acquisition phase. During this period, the patient's

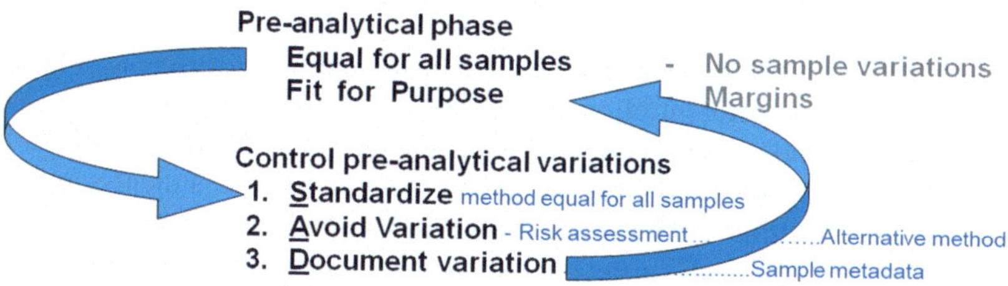

Fig. 4.2 Controlling sample variation in the pre-analytical phase (1) standardize the entire workflow, if a step in the workflow cannot be standardized, (2) try to avoid the chosen method by performing a risk analysis, if it is not possible to avoid the method, then (3) document the variations in the method or step. The documentation of the variations generates sample metadata which can be used as tool for identification and control of sample variation and self-improvement

well-being has of course the highest priority and brings in many variants as described earlier that cannot be standardized. Where important variations cannot be eliminated by standardization, the next best approach is to try to avoid the activity causing the variation (see Fig. 4.2). This can be done by performing a risk assessment. However, this option may not be readily applicable for many of the variants that are introduced. Another approach is to use a test that is not sensitive to the introduced variation. However, this is not an option if the analytical technique is too sensitive. The last option is then to record or document the actions that can cause sample variation suspected of influencing gene expression, protein modification, metabolism, and decay of proteins, RNA, and DNA. This means that (meta-) data needs to be recorded during the pre-acquisition phase of the tissue sample on the treatment or intervention, and how it is performed. Parameters that can have such influence are, e.g.:

- Warm ischemic time: The time point where the blood supply of organs is cut off or disturbed until the time point where the organ is removed from the body are used to calculate the duration of the warm ischemic period.
- Type of surgical tools used (can enhance decay of macromolecules).
- Medication/drugs given during, just before as well as before the tissue was taken from the body (depending on the drug's influence span).
- General condition of the patient and his/her concomitant diseases.
- Cold ischemic time: The time point of the removal of the tissue from the body and the time point of preservation (freezing of fixation) are needed to calculate this period.
- Temperature or cooling of the tissues during transport.
- Genetic background.
- Lifestyle and environment.

These parameters can be used in two ways: (1) Cohort selection, where parameters of known influences on the test, can be chosen to have a limited maximum or minimum value; (2) Recognize outliers during analysis of the test. The parameter values can be used to determine whether a sample is fit for purpose, or not, in the selection of a new batch for the same test (see Fig. 4.2). The variants introduced during the pre-acquisition phase can also result in significant differences between samples collected in different clinical centers. Therefore, in multicenter research projects which include tissues collected for research, it can be very worthwhile to engage all involved clinicians (e.g., surgeons, pathologists, treatment specialists) from all involved institutes in the study design and analysis, where they can discuss differences in their approach during the intervention. Some of the differences might then be easily resolved upfront.

4.4 Tissue Collecting Environments

Tissues can be collected in the diagnostic pathway either with or without a clinical request for pathology diagnosis. The source of tissue specimens or biopsies can be located in the operating room, the outpatient clinics, and the pathology morgue, resulting in surgical specimens, (needle) biopsies, and postmortem materials, respectively. Surgical specimens or biopsies with a clinical request for diagnostic pathology always need to be evaluated by a pathologist having the legal responsibility for the diagnostic process. Moreover, a tissue is not homogenous, otherwise you could call the tissue sample an aliquot instead of a sample. A tumor for instance can harbor a small aggressive tumor type that may not be missed in the diagnosis. Therefore, the pathologist needs to inspect and evaluate the specimen in the state as it was removed from the body, before samples may be taken from the specimen for research purposes. This is required in order not to disturb the primary clinical responsibility, which is the diagnostic process, with a secondary interest, medical research. Therefore, surgical specimens with a clinical request for diagnostic pathology need to be transported to an area where the pathologist can perform his macro analysis on the intact surgical specimen, and decide what parts of the fresh tissue are not needed for diagnostic purposes and can be spared for the frozen tissue bank. It can happen that the macro protocols demand all available tissue for microscopic evaluation and nothing can be spared for the frozen tissue bank. After the samples are taken, the remaining tissue can be fixed in buffered formalin to be sampled for diagnosis later. Tissues without further diagnostic requests can be sampled and preserved without pathology inspection and preserved on-site in the location where they are removed from the body.

4.4.1 Pathology Archive

Only small fragments of tissue are needed for microscopic evaluation of tissue morphologic characteristics for diagnostic purposes. The best images for microscopic evaluation are obtained from FFPE tissue fragments. Therefore, the pathologists sample smaller fragments from the formalin-fixed surgical specimen with a maximum size of 3 × 2 × 0.5 cm at strategic sites important for diagnosis and described in macro protocols, for further microscopic evaluation. Postmortem material is usually collected in the approximate size of fragments suitable for microscopic analysis, whereas biopsies are collected in smaller sizes and often almost all material needs to be evaluated for diagnosis. These fragments are usually embedded in paraffin to form blocks that can easily be cut into microscopic sections. Only small parts of the fragments are used for the microscopic evaluation. The remainder of the fragments are routinely preserved and kept after diagnosis at the pathology laboratory and serve a legal purpose as part of the documentation of the given diagnosis. Pathology departments usually are obligated by law to keep this documentation for decades. The duration differs by country due to differences in local regulations. The tissue fragments are preserved as FFPE blocks, stained glass slides, or as frozen tissue. These archives contain a wealth of information that has been shown to be very beneficial for medical research discoveries. The tissues can be used for medical research, but their primary diagnostic purpose cannot be forgotten in the process. Therefore, samples may not be depleted. The original lesion must be preserved for possible later use. The archive seems very attractive because the collection is already there in massive numbers and very well documented in terms of disease, diagnosis, and follow-up. However, it must be considered that derivatives like DNA, RNA, and proteins may not always be available in an acceptable quality due to the fixation processes. Although this approach may appear to be standardized from the outside, because almost all pathology labs use buffered formalin nowadays, there are still many variations allowed in the collection and fixation processes. However, the time and the duration the tissue is fixed vary a lot even within one lab. Tissues that arrive in the lab on Monday, Tuesday, and Wednesday are fixed in formalin for about 36–44 h, whereas tissues arriving Tuesday and Friday are fixed for much longer periods, due to the weekend, and fixation can last for 60–84 h. However, a shorter fixation of about 24 h would preserve RNA and DNA better. For the larger surgical specimen, the penetration rate becomes an issue. The inside of a tissue is fixed over a longer time period than the outside. For this reason, larger specimens are randomly cut just before fixation to allow the formalin to penetrate the tissues faster, whereas hollow ones need to be opened so as not to form air bubbles. Also, due to practical reasons, larger specimens are not always fixed in the optimal tissue to volume ratio. Despite all these variations the diagnostic tests seem to give solid stable results. The reason is that the pathology tests are designed, validated, and selected to be insensitive to these particular variations. Theoretically, this is again a perfect example for the second option in the schema given in Fig. 4.2, i.e., where standardization is not possible the variation can be avoided by choosing an insensitive test. The molecular diagnostic tests can in most cases be adapted in such a way they can use FFPE tissues as input material. The tests used for research are sometimes improved or innovated in a manner where it is indeed possible to use FFPE as input material. However, awareness of a large amount of possible variations and even chemical changes is needed for the choice of the sample. Further details are described in another chapter of this book.

4.4.2 Fresh Frozen Tissue

As an alternative, tissues can be frozen. This way the formalin chemical, ratio, duration, and penetration effects are avoided. In addition, DNA, RNA, proteins, and metabolites are preserved in a much more native state. Frozen tissues can therefore be used in highly sensitive tests, where the quality of the extracted derivatives plays a more pronounced role. Freezing is often seen as the golden standard.

It is important to strive to freeze the samples within 30 min after the tissue is removed from the body. Therefore, the freezing process must be relatively fast. To speed up the process, the vials should be prelabeled. The label should carry a bar code and readable text. The tissues received for freezing should have a bar coded label carrying the pathology number and/or patient number. This way the bar codes can be scanned into the database of a tracking program or the patient label can be adhered to a form on which the vial numbers are taken over. Then the tissue specifics like the tissue type (e.g., colon, kidney, lung, etc.), disease state of the tissue (e.g., tumor/affected, unaffected, metastasis, inflammatory, infection, etc.), estimated size, time of freezing, and SOP deviations are entered into the database of a sample tracking system or in the form related to the correct vial number. To populate the database in a coherent and reusable way the data entry pages should make use of file management tools such as Dropbox or radio buttons whenever possible. The vial should be carefully chosen to fit adequately in the storage system, i.e., not wasting space. Large vials are mostly not used to capacity and large portions of tissue can be cut to smaller fragments, resulting in more aliquots. This way space is used more efficiently, and having more samples leaves non-manipulated spare ones for other experiments. Storage systems in columns can be consolidated within the freezer, fitting the available space efficiently to capacity. As an alternative, tissue samples can be taken from a surgical specimen using a biopsy needle and transfer the biopsy into a straw for freezing in liquid nitrogen [6].

For reasons of the orientation of the tissue sample, the tissue can be frozen placed on a piece cut to size of thin layered cork under a Whatman paper cut to approximately the same size and moistened with a physiologic salt solution. The tissue is placed on top and quickly frozen together, preferably snap frozen in precooled isopentane ≤ -80 °C.

For the diagnostic freezing process itself, good morphology is very important for the analysis by the pathologist and can contribute to the analysis of the medical research results. Frozen tissue slides have an inferior morphology compared to tissue slides derived from FFPE. Using a snap freezing process, where in this typical example the tissue fragment of about 1–3 cm^3 is placed in precooled isopentane (C_5H_{12}, methylbutane or 2-methylbutane) with a temperature between or equal to -80 °C and -160 °C, freezes the tissue almost instantly, without causing a lot of damage to the tissue. Slower freezing processes like flash freezing, e.g., putting tissue in a vial and storing in a -80 °C freezer or submerging it with or without a vial directly into liquid nitrogen can damage the tissue morphology. Tissues can be damaged by crystal formation and rising salt concentrations within the cells due to the withdrawal of water by the freezing process. The rising salt concentration can cause cell lysis. Freezing the tissue very fast does not allow these processes to show much effect. Directly placing a sample in liquid nitrogen (−196 °C) seems very effective however the liquid nitrogen immediately starts to boil and the gas phase nitrogen surrounding the sample forms an insulating layer not capable of transferring the heat fast enough from the sample. This is called the Leidenfrost effect [7]. Precooled isopentane is used to avoid the Leidenfrost effect [7]. It has a different boiling temperature and stays liquid during the freezing process, and can rapidly transfer the warmth from the sample to the surrounding liquid. Precooling isopentane until it is below −80 °C (in liquid nitrogen or dry ice) can readily snap freeze the tissue sample. When precooling with liquid nitrogen, care must be taken not to freeze the isopentane. It freezes at −160 °C but becomes opaque at −150 °C. Hanging the opaque isopentane container just above the liquid nitrogen keeps it in the proper temperature range for a long time (Fig. 4.3). For cooling to −80 °C, a tube with isopentane can be put in dry ice, or special cooling units are available which have a convenient small space that can be filled with isopentane cooled to −80 °C, and a surrounding environment of −40 °C where samples can be accumulated for storage at the end of the day. Results have been published on a limited number of tissue types and samples showing good morphology after freezing without precooled isopentane in liquid nitrogen on the bottom of a precooled aluminum vial [8]. However, these results could not be reproduced during the validation of this method with more samples and tissue types in the hands of routine personnel (unpublished results). The method under validation involved too many variables in daily practice.

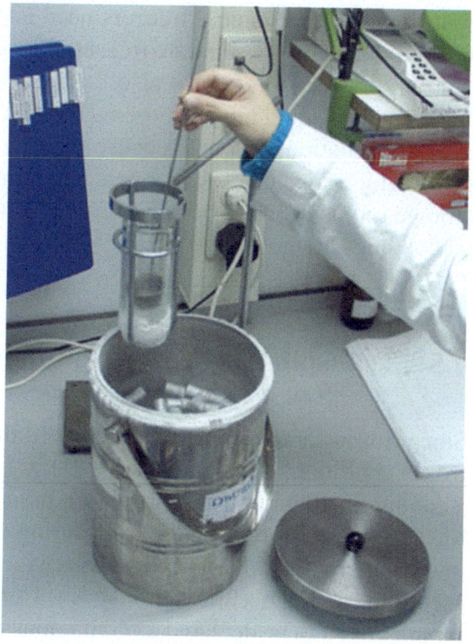

Fig. 4.3 Example of a precooled isopentane set-up in daily practice

After (snap) freezing the tissue it is transferred to its precooled vial and must be kept frozen throughout its further existence as a sample. Due to the freezing process, the cell membranes are damaged and the cell compartments no longer separated. This can release proteins responsible for the decay of other proteins, RNA, and metabolites in direct contact, which is not possible during the living state. For instance, RNA is degraded in a short time after thawing tissues, especially frozen tissue slides, where the cells are even further damaged by the cutting process. This instability of RNA in tissue that has been frozen is also the reason why RNA quality can be used as a quality indicator in a quality control program. It can be used to test SOP adherence and even indicate freezer failure where collections have been thawed.

4.4.3 Fresh Frozen Tissue Storage

A complete overview concerning the demands of sample storage in tissue banks has been described in published best practices and guidelines [1–5]. Here, only the most important issues are presented. For long-term storage, the frozen tissue samples must be stored at a temperature below −70 °C (−80 °C freezer) [1–5]. The collections are valuable and need to be protected against thawing or uncontrolled handling. Storage systems need to be equipped with alarm systems that warn personnel trained to handle system failures especially during the night, weekends, and holidays. There are many different storage systems available, each with its own advantages and disadvantages. Backup capacity needs to be available and ready to use when freezers break down or when the cooling units in freezer rooms fail. Rooms with separate mechanical freezers need adequate cooling systems to dissipate the heat produced by the separate freezer units. Emergency power needs to be available not only for the freezers but also for the cooling systems dissipating the heat from the freezers. Liquid nitrogen rooms need oxygen alarm systems connected to emergency ventilation systems because the evaporated nitrogen can cause low oxygen levels which are dangerous for personnel. In general, the safety of the location of the storage rooms needs to be considered, and they need to be safe from disasters such as flooding (basements) or fire.

4.5 Transport of Frozen Samples

Since frozen samples may not be thawed during transport, they must be shipped in frozen condition. Usually dry ice (−80 °C) or liquid nitrogen (−196 °C) are used as a cooling medium to transport frozen tissue samples. These are preferentially used for short-term storage in the lab during handling of the samples. For transport involving couriers, the samples and refrigerant must be packaged and documented according to IATA (International Air Transport Association) rules, where frozen samples need to be declared as contagious materials. Special containers, labels, and documents are available for transport, and the courier can be asked to regularly monitor the amount of dry ice or liquid nitrogen and refill when levels become low. The temperature during long-term transport can be monitored using small devices that can record the exact temperature during the transport. Shipments should not be planned in such a way that frozen samples arrive on Friday or on weekends.

4.6 Fresh Frozen Tissue Quality Optimization

4.6.1 Quality Control and Quality Assurance

A typical quality control program for SOP adherence would involve checking randomly 1–2% of the new samples for RNA quality, correct placement in the storage system, the right number according to the administration in the right place and the right type of tissue with the expected disease state. To check the latter, it is necessary to prepare a frozen H&E tissue slide, which is evaluated by a pathologist. Determination of the RNA Integrity Number (RIN) value is typically used for these quality checks. However, other and more reliable methods like determination of the RNA Ct values can also be used [9]. A RIN value of >6.5 can be considered as good quality that is fit for purpose for most techniques [10]. A random method will also bring in samples that are known for bad quality RNA because the tissue only has a small amount of RNA or a very high RNAse content, e.g., fatty or squamous tissue, pancreatic tissue, or necrotic tissue (which should be avoided to enter the collection). For this reason, an initial 20% of RNA samples with quality not meeting the threshold is not unusual. In addition, individual RNA extractions might be false negative and warrant repeating the extraction. Especially those samples that show a bad RNA quality but a good morphology have a fair chance to perform better when the extraction is repeated. In the situation where the amount of RNA quality falls below 20%, plans should be made to carefully inspect SOP adherence and look for possible interpretation errors under the existing SOPs.

Some tissue banks perform quality control on the sample content shortly after collection. This can be done in several ways. One approach is to take a fragment of the tissue to be frozen and place it in a cassette for further FFPE preparation, followed by H&E staining of a tissue slide. This can only be done with samples large enough to spare material for this separate preparation. Another method is to prepare a frozen H&E tissue slide directly from every sample. The disadvantage of this approach is that the sample preferably needs to be mounted using OCT or Tissue Tek. This substance can be however very harmful for any future proteomics work and small amounts contaminate the tissue slides taken for proteomics testing. If this method is used, only very small amounts of OCT must be applied, and only at the bottom of the frozen tissue sample. There are also alternatives on the market that do not show this effect [11].

Accreditation or certification of the tissue bank is very beneficial for the assurance of quality. Regular audits and the necessity of having standard procedures in place improve the existing quality and services. For a tissue bank to function well it needs dedicated and competent personnel, who are involved in all the typical biobanking processes. These processes can be perfectly controlled and improved where necessary within an accreditation or certification program. An increasing number of pathology departments worldwide have become accredited under ISO 15189 or a similar accreditation program. A tissue bank can also seek accreditation for ISO 20387. Such standards are however general. For specific applications, there are specific technical standards that contain norms and information for specific techniques or workflows [12]. Useful examples for tissue are ISO 20184-1 and 2 that describe Molecular in vitro diagnostic examinations—Specifications for preexamination processes for frozen tissue—Part 1 Isolated RNA and Part 2 Isolated proteins. ISO 20166-1, 2, and 3 also cover the preexamination but for FFPE tissues and isolated RNA, protein, and DNA, respectively.

Due to the integration of frozen tissue banks in the diagnostic pathways of pathology departments, they are obliged to coordinate their SOPs under the accreditation of the ISO 15189, with the beneficial regime of audits and improvement processes.

Proficiency Testing (PT) and External Quality Assurance (EQA), where the biobank's competence is compared with other laboratories, are essential for harmonization of quality. PT testing is offered for biobanking, including tissue banks, for several tests concerning several end products.

Although the existing guidelines, best practices, minimal standards for biobanking, general accreditation like ISO 20387/ISO15189, certification ISO9001, etc., referred to in this chapter have a harmonizing effect, the laboratories harboring tissue banks still have many choices for methods at their disposal. Such differences need to be considered when exchanging frozen samples for multicenter research projects using sensitive tests. Information concerning the clinical part of the pre-acquisition phase also needs to be included. Specific ISO standards like the technical standards ISO 20166 and ISO 20184 can increase reproducibility by introducing norms for the pre-analytical phase in specific circumstances [12] to collect sample metadata that can be used as a tool for identification and control of sample variation. The tool can be used to see if samples are fit for purpose and to increase the laboratory or biobank performance in both diagnostics and research [12].

4.6.2 *Optimization of the Pre-Acquisition Phase*

It is known that RNA and protein expression patterns can vary due to warm ischemic time [13, 14]. The influence of cold ischemic (below body temperature) time has also been observed [15–21]. However, the effect of extra cooling after removal from the body between 4 °C and 0 °C (on ice) [3] can delay such effects [13, 16]. Artifacts in expression or molecular changes can already be observed after 30 min at room temperature [15]. Although there are still matters under debate on this point, it is good to strive for freezing within 30 min after the surgical specimen has been removed from the body. The warm and cold ischemic times, as well as the cold ischemic temperature, should be recorded and added to the sample data as metadata. When small biopsies are transported, it is best to keep them in a dry small tightly closed container cooled on ice and freeze them as fast as possible to avoid loss of morphology and minimize variability of gene expression [16]. Tissues can be stabilized in plastic bags under vacuum and at 0–4 °C during transport and promotes the stabilization of RNA and proteins. This procedure allows not only the collection of frozen samples for biobanks but also routine microscopic evaluation [22].

4.6.3 Tissue Sources and Quality

Tissues from surgical specimens collected in the proper way can have a very high quality and be very useful for medical research. The quality of DNA, RNA, proteins, and metabolites is close to the native state in living cells, and if the tissue is frozen fast enough the expression/concentration/levels resemble closely the living state. However, the influence of warm ischemic time, cold ischemic time, or surgery-related effects (drugs, wound trauma, or surgical tools) might cause a bias in the end result.

Biopsies have a very useful characteristic in avoiding variations introduced in the pre-analytical phase of a surgical specimen [23]. Biopsies have almost no warm ischemic time effects and if frozen instantly, almost no cold ischemic time. They are however a lot more difficult to obtain because for the patient it is a very intrusive method. In addition, biopsies are small and can mostly not be used both for diagnostics and research purposes. In addition, most biopsies will be used routinely for microscopic evaluation and stored as FFPE material. That means they are not available as frozen residual tissues and separate biopsies need to be taken for research purposes. This needs to be very well augmented for METC or IRB approval because the same material might be readily available for the study from residual diagnostic material in the pathology archive.

Postmortem samples are also frozen however due to the long warm and cold ischemic effects, the advanced decay process of macromolecules can become an issue for many analyses [24]. Although these samples can be useful, they will not always qualify to be fit for purpose.

4.7 Using Frozen Tissue Samples

4.7.1 Extraction of Derivatives

Frozen samples should never be allowed to thaw during manipulation. If this happens all RNA is degraded. In addition, proteins can interact outside their normal compartments with other proteins, macromolecules, and metabolites. This can be accomplished when preparing frozen tissue slides at −20 °C for derivative extraction, and after the slides have been cut immediately put the sample in −80 °C or a lower temperature environment. In case the sample thaws in the process, it must not be returned to the biobank. To check for possible effects of tissue heterogeneity, it is advised to take out a tissue slide from the top and one after the fifth or tenth slide used for extraction, perform H&E staining, and ask the pathologist to evaluate the tissue contents of both slides. Keep the glass slides or images of the slides for documentation.

For RNA extraction, ideally the tissue slides are immediately submerged in the frozen state in the extraction buffer (only use tools cooled to −20 °C, but do not cool the extraction buffer). Sometimes it is necessary to (laser) micro dissect tissues to avoid influences caused by tissue heterogeneity. There are protocols that allow RNA extraction after laser microdissection at room temperature. These protocols usually mildly fix the still frozen tissue slide in cold alcohol followed by cold dehydration and staining.

4.7.2 Tissue Research Support

For medical research, it can be very beneficial to make use of the knowledge and routines of a pathology department. Pathology expertise can be especially important to evaluate the heterogeneity of tissues and can be crucial to the quality of the anticipated results. Pathologists can help in the determination of those cells contributing to the actual diagnosis. Pathologists can also offer expertise in techniques that are focused on tissue, such as tissue laser microdissection and tissue microarrays. However, offering simple, embedding, freezing, cutting, or staining techniques in combination with special stains and molecular diagnostics can markedly improve the research results. In addition, offering these techniques under ISO conditions guarantees a certain quality level for not only scientists in the institute, but also for companies performing medical research who often need their suppliers to be certified or accredited as well. Moreover, following the ISO technical standards would even contribute to the general reproducibility of results as well as compliance to new European regulations for In Vitro Diagnostic tests [12, 25]. Another even more important point is that the unique material collected in the tissue bank is used optimally, leading to results important for the patients, who expect productive results from their altruistic donation.

Acknowledgment Much of the work presented here was discovered or created within the European Union FP7 project SPIDIA (contract no. 222916), the European Union's Horizon 2020 project SPIDIA4P (contract no. 733112), and the FP7 project EUROCANPLATFORM (contract no. 260791). We thank all the project coordinators and partners for their support and discussions.

References

1. OECD (ed) (2007) OECD best practice guidelines for biological resource centers—general best practice guidelines for all BRCs. OECD, Paris. http://www.oecd.org/dataoecd/7/13/38777417.pdf. Accessed March 2015
2. OECD (ed) (2009) Guidelines on human biobanks and genetic research databases. OECD, Paris. http://www.oecd.org/dataoecd/41/47/44054609.pdf. Accessed March 2015
3. International Society for Biological and Environmental Repositories (ISBER) (2012) Best practices for repositories: collection, storage, retrieval and distribution of biological materials for research. Biopreserv Biobank 10:79–161
4. NCI best practices for specimen resources. NCI, Bethesda. 2007. http://biospecimens.cancer.gov/global/pdfs/NCI_Best_Practices_060507.pdf. Accessed March 2015
5. Caboux E, Plymoth A, Hainaut P (eds) (2007) International network of biological resource centres for cancer research: recommendations on common minimal technical standards. IARC/WHO, Lyon
6. Morente MM, Mager R, Alonso S et al (2006) TuBaFrost 2: standardising tissue collection and quality control procedures for a European virtual frozen tissue bank network. Eur J Cancer 42:2684–2691
7. Peters SR (2010) A practical guide to frozen section technique. Springer, New York. e-isbn:978-1-4419-1234-3
8. Mager SR, Oomen MH, Morente MM et al (2007) Standard operating procedure for the collection of fresh frozen tissue samples. Eur J Cancer 43:828–834
9. Kashofer K, Viertler C, Pichler M et al (2013) Quality control of RNA preservation and extraction from paraffin-embedded tissue: implications for RT-PCR and microarray analysis. PLoS One 8(7):e70714. https://doi.org/10.1371/journal.pone.0070714
10. Kap M, Oomen M, Arshad S, de Jong B, Riegman P (2014) Fit for purpose frozen tissue collections by RNA integrity number-based quality control assurance at the Erasmus MC tissue bank. Biopreserv Biobank 12:81–90. https://doi.org/10.1089/bio.2013.0051
11. Snijders MLH, Zajec M, Walter LAJ et al (2019) Cryo-gel embedding compound for renal biopsy biobanking. Sci Rep 9:15250. https://doi.org/10.1038/s41598-019-51962-8
12. Riegman PHJ, Becker KF, Zatloukal K et al (2019) How standardization of the pre-analytical phase of both research and diagnostic biomaterials can increase reproducibility of biomedical research and diagnostics. New Biotechnol 53:35–40. https://doi.org/10.1016/j.nbt.2019.06.007
13. Gündisch S, Annaratone L, Beese C et al (2015) Critical roles of specimen type and temperature before and during fixation in the detection of phosphoproteins in breast cancer tissues. Lab Invest. 95(5):561–571. https://doi.org/10.1038/labinvest.2015.37
14. Gündisch S, Hauck S, Sarioglu H et al (2012) Variability of protein and phosphoprotein levels in clinical tissue specimens during the preanalytical phase. J Proteome Res 11:5748–5762. https://doi.org/10.1021/pr300560y
15. Spruessel A, Steimann G, Jung M et al (2004) Tissue ischemia time affects gene and protein expression patterns within minutes following surgical tumor excision. Biotechniques 36:1030–1037
16. Kap M, Sieuwerts AM, Kubista M et al (2015) The influence of tissue procurement procedures on RNA integrity, gene expression and morphology in porcine and human liver tissue. Biopreserv Biobank 13(3):200–206

17. David KA, Unger FT, Uhlig P et al (2014) Surgical procedures and postsurgical tissue processing significantly affect expression of genes and EGFR-pathway proteins in colorectal cancer tissue. Oncotarget 5:11017–11028
18. Ma Y, Dai H, Kong X (2012) Impact of warm ischemia on gene expression analysis in surgically removed biosamples. Anal Biochem 423:229–235. https://doi.org/10.1016/j.ab.2012.02.003
19. Dash A, Maine IP, Varambally S et al (2002) Changes in differential gene expression because of warm ischemia time of radical prostatectomy specimens. Am J Pathol 161:1743–1748
20. Huang J, Qi R, Quackenbush J, Dauway E et al (2002) Effects of ischemia on gene expression. J Surg Res 99:222–227
21. de Cremoux P, Valet F, Gentien D et al (2011) Importance of pre-analytical steps for transcriptome and RT-qPCR analyses in the context of the phase II randomised multicentre trial REMAGUS02 of neoadjuvant chemotherapy in breast cancer patients. BMC Cancer 11:215. https://doi.org/10.1186/1471-2407-11-215
22. Di Novi C, Minniti D, Barbaro S et al (2010) Sci Total Environ 408:3092–3095
23. Basik M, Aguilar-Mahecha A, Rousseau C et al (2013) Biopsies: next-generation biospecimens for tailoring therapy. Nat Rev Clin Oncol 10:437–450. https://doi.org/10.1038/nrclinonc.2013.101
24. van der Linden A, Blokker BM, Kap M et al (2014) Post-mortem tissue biopsies obtained at minimally invasive autopsy: an RNA-quality analysis. PLoS One 9:e115675. https://doi.org/10.1371/journal.pone.0115675
25. Dagher G, Becker KF, Bonin S, Foy C, Gelmini S, Kubista M, Kungl P, Oelmueller U, Parkes H, Pinzani P, Riegman P, Schröder U, Stumptner C, Turano P, Sjöback R, Wutte A, Zatloukal K (2019) Pre-analytical processes in medical diagnostics: New regulatory requirements and standards. N Biotechnol 52:121–125. https://doi.org/10.1016/j.nbt.2019.05.002. Epub 2019 May 15. PMID: 31102798.

Chapter 5
The Use of Paraffin Blocks/Pathology Archives for Clinical Biobanking

Giorgio Stanta and Serena Bonin

Abstract Every human tissue collected from surgery or biopsy is formalin-fixed and paraffin-embedded (FFPE). A huge quantity of human tissues is preserved in hospitals, and it is possible to estimate that in Europe about three hundred million new specimens of tissues are stored in archives every year. These archive tissues (AT) represent any type of even rare pathological lesions with a number of cases sufficient for any possible study. Frequent evidence of acquired resistance to the new targeted therapies has posed clinicians new issues to be addressed, such as the need to go back to patients' tissues. Increasingly more often we have to use ATs because of clinical research, which is now starting to be an integrated process with applied medicine. We cannot separate clinics from clinical research, it is a unique entity. This creates new necessities such as better quality ATs, more standardized methods, a careful choice of the tissues, and a better organization. The pathology archives of hospitals are clinical biorepositories that are different from a research biobank. The major difference is related to the clinical purpose of these archives; even though this may not seem to be an obstacle to their utilization for research purposes, it is perfectly fitted with the most recent necessities of a kind of clinical research that is strictly related to medicine and perfectly integrated into it. The use of AT biorepositories represents a peculiar type of tissue as a source that also needs a different bioethical approach.

Keywords Biobank · Formalin-fixed and paraffin-embedded tissues · Network · Pathology · Clinical research

5.1 Introduction

Every human tissue collected from surgery or biopsy is formalin-fixed and paraffin-embedded (FFPE). A huge quantity of human tissues is preserved in hospitals, and it is possible to estimate that in Europe about three hundred million new specimens of

---

G. Stanta (✉) · S. Bonin
Department of Medical Sciences, University of Trieste, Cattinara University Hospital, Trieste, Italy
e-mail: stanta@impactsnetwork.eu; sbonin@units.it

P. Hainaut et al. (eds.), *Biobanking of Human Biospecimens*,
https://doi.org/10.1007/978-3-030-55901-4_5

tissues are stored in archives every year. These archive tissues (AT) represent any type of even rare pathological lesions with a number of cases sufficient for any possible study. Frequent evidence of acquired resistance to the new targeted therapies has posed clinicians new issues to be addressed, such as the need to go back to patients' tissues. Increasingly we have to use ATs because of clinical research, which is now starting to be an integrated process with applied medicine. We cannot separate clinics from clinical research, it is a unique entity. This creates new necessities such as better quality ATs, more standardized methods, a careful choice of the tissues, and a better organization. The pathology archives of hospitals are clinical biorepositories that are different from a research biobank. The major difference is related to the clinical purpose of these archives; even though this may not seem to be an obstacle to their utilization for research purposes, it is perfectly fitted with the most recent necessities of a kind of clinical research that is strictly related to medicine and perfectly integrated into it. The use of AT biorepositories represents a peculiar type of tissue as a source that also needs a different bioethical approach.

5.2 Archive Tissues

Every human tissue collected for clinical reasons, from surgery or biopsy or even of autopsy origin, is formalin-fixed and paraffin-embedded (FFPE). After few sections are cut for diagnostic purposes, the remaining tissues are stored, sometimes for decades, in the pathology archives of hospitals; for this reason, they are called archive tissues (AT). The time these ATs are stored varies from country to country, from few years to over 20 years, but on average in Europe they are stored for 10 years, and in some academic institutions even forever. This means that a huge quantity of human tissues is preserved in hospitals, and it is possible to estimate that in Europe about three hundred million new specimens of tissues from clinical activities are stored in archives every year. These ATs represent any type of even rare pathological lesions or rare subtypes of common entities, with a number of cases sufficient for any possible clinical study. Interest in performing molecular analyses in these tissues is not only related to clinical research, but above all to the fact that they are the only tissues available from patients, and today they are frequently used for molecular diagnostics. Therefore, we are more interested than ever in performing high-quality level molecular analyses in ATs.

Molecular medicine, or better today's precision medicine [1], takes new necessities that today are an integral part of medicine into the clinical practice. We know that research is strictly related to applied medicine with a continuous translational activity of information from basic research to clinics; this is a long process that needs a lot of technical, clinical, and bioethical precautions. This process starts from cell cultures and animal models, to continue then with clinical tissues coming from biobank networks that can provide high-quality fresh-frozen tissues with related clinical information. The last step for any verified and validated biomarker is the use of FFPE tissues of patients to reach a diffused clinical utilization. However, routinely performed analysis in patients is not the final step of the process. Recently, frequent evidence of acquired resistance to the new targeted therapies has posed

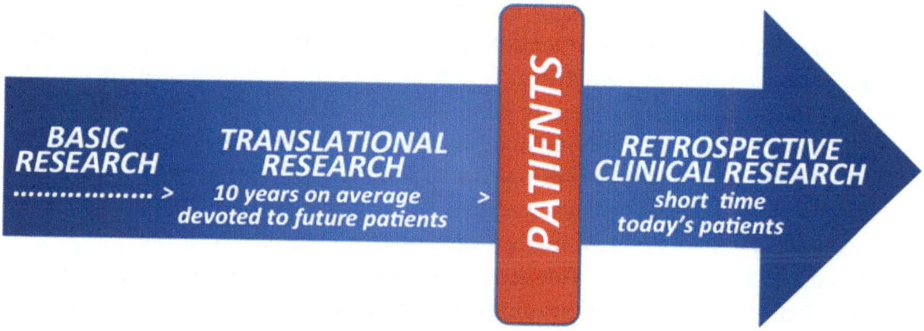

Fig. 5.1 Relationship between basic, translational, and retrospective clinical research by time and clinical application

clinicians new issues to be addressed such as the need to go back to patients' tissues to study the molecular substrate of these events. Increasingly we have to use ATs because of clinical research, which is now starting to be an integrated process with applied medicine. We cannot separate clinics from clinical research, it is a unique entity. This creates new necessities such as better quality ATs, more standardized and controlled research methods, a careful choice of the tissues to be analyzed (see tumor heterogeneity) [2], but also a new approach to bioethics because this process is not separated from applied medicine, but it is strictly part of it (Fig. 5.1).

Awareness of immediate clinical utility and application of new specific discoveries in this field also make it necessary to set up new tissue networks. Clinical research can be improved indeed by the possibility to rapidly organize research with a sufficient number of cases, which cannot be available in a single institution especially for less frequent subtypes, or for rapid verification and validation of clinical biomarkers [3]. This is extremely important not only for future clinical use but in particular to be applied to today's patients with a continuous update. The need for organized networks was recently recognized by the European biobank infrastructure (BBMRI-ERIC) [4], which started to study the organization of an AT biobanking network with the activities of an "Archive Tissue Working Group." This initiative has already started in Italy with NIPAB (Network of Italian Pathology Archive Biobanks), which is part of the Italian node BBMRI-IT [5].

5.3 Pathology Archives

The pathology archives of hospitals are clinical biorepositories that, for this reason, are different from a research biobank even if the sources of human tissues are the same. The major difference is related to the clinical purpose of these archives; even though this may seem to be an obstacle to their utilization for research purposes, it is perfectly fitted with the most recent necessities of a kind of clinical research that is strictly related to medicine and perfectly integrated into it. It represents a type of clinical biobank of ATs specific for this kind of clinical research. Anyway, this is not something new because since Virchow, in the second half of the nineteenth century, collection and study of such tissues have taken to modern medicine, with the continued recognition of new and better defined clinical entities. This has recently taken to outstanding results by Juan Rosai [6]. Now that DNA human sequences have been revealed and the new concept of precision medicine is starting to be developed, we have to tackle new phenotypic and heterogeneous complexities; again clinical tissues are essential for the definition of the new medical taxonomy [1]. Recently liquid biopsies as circulating tumor cells (CTC) or circulating free DNA (cfDNA) have been analyzed with a great interest especially for cases of recurrent cancer, but still the real meaning of this evidence must be understood. In addition, the major clinical interest is to treat primary tumors even in cases in which clinically undetected spread is already active. This means that tissues are still at the center of clinical research. Primary tumors have to reveal the entire intra-tumor heterogeneous genetic, epigenetic, and the homo- and heterotypic phenotype landscape, which now seems to have rather an "organoid" pattern than a simple collection of cells. Only this complexity in primary and metastatic cancer tissues can show the real functional mechanism of cancer and give opportunities to avoid clinical recurrences better than simply trying to control them.

5.4 Utility of AT Biobanks Network

The use of AT biorepositories represents a peculiar type of tissue as source, analysis methodology, and bioethical approach. The idea to define them as a special type of biobank and to include them in the European biobank infrastructure (BBMRI-ERIC) [4] was developed for many reasons. Pathology archives have already been organized to absolve their clinical function of reserves of clinical tissues which can be reused for further diagnostic procedures and as a source of clinical information for the patients also as a legal base. When we switch to clinical research, there is the obligation to maintain the previous clinical functions as a primary goal, but also to reach a new level of coordination and efficiency for the needs of clinical research. The inclusion in a European infrastructure level (BBMRI_ERIC), based on country nodes as reference centers of the single institution, can supply clinical research with common rules and services to produce a more effective network. In this way, better access to major case studies for rare entities or rare subtypes of common pathologies is provided. The network can also give useful feedback for diagnostics with technical improvement in the pre-analytical quality of tissues, in standardization and reproducibility of analytical methods, in the selection of tissues to be analyzed to avoid the effects of heterogeneity and in providing clinical information of better quality [3].

The consequences can be highly relevant for medicine; they include acceleration of clinical research, rapid verification and validation of clinical biomarkers (especially those related to intrinsic and acquired resistance), verification of clinical cases, efficacy of the new therapies, therapy response subgroups, very long follow-up studies, treatment performance evaluation and assessment of costs and benefits.

Table 5.1 Summary of the advantages of AT biobanking network in a European infrastructure

Box 1: Why including A.T. biobanking network in a European infrastructure?
To take collections of archive tissues to a new level of coordination and efficiency for clinical research
To provide new common services for the community of archive tissue biobanks
To contribute to the pan-European research infrastructure BBMRI-ERIC
To support and accelerate clinical research (e.g., identifying and validating new biomarkers and causes of acquired resistance)
To harmonize the collection of samples of specific rare diseases or rare subtypes of common lesions
To test the efficacy of the new therapies and therapy response subgroups with established costs and benefits
To improve the pre-analytical quality of tissues, the standardization and reproducibility of analytical methods and the selection of tissues to be analyzed to avoid the drawbacks of heterogeneity
To allow access to developed fully established ELSI platform

All these activities are essential for a new medicine on the way of "precision medicine." This network will facilitate the connection between biobanks and then with clinical organizations by standardization and harmonization of activities, and with industry that can rapidly better orient new drugs useful for patients as summarized in Table 5.1.

5.5 Bioethical Specificity of AT Clinical Research

A basic requirement for this new biobank network is to adapt bioethical rules to their activities, which are quite different from those of traditional biobanks, with access to a fully established ELSI platform. Specificities are related to the fact that, first of all, this is not just research but today it is a clinical activity strictly connected with practical medicine and that new medicine cannot be performed without it. The second point is that the actors are part of the practical clinical process; pathologists, oncologists, etc., are involved in the diagnostic/treatment process and for this reason they are subjected to professional secrecy, which in every country is more restrictive than any privacy rule. The legal consequences of any infraction are very severe, with a high level of guarantee. Third, there is a direct interest in the patients, because the consequences of this type of clinical research can directly influence the donor patients and not just future patients with an average time gap of 10 years, as in translational medicine. The bioethical question is still open and unresolved in most European countries, most of all because the specificity of this kind of activity has not been recognized. We absolutely need a wide discussion at the European level, with the participation of the major medical organizations and societies, and also with patients' associations. A common European directive could be important for an effective practical approach to the issue.

5.6 How to Organize the Network?

The network has been set up as a virtual network of pathology archives that are devoted to clinical activities (Table 5.2). These archives are usually arranged by biopsy number, and related to clinical information sufficient to complete the diagnostic process. Today they are often correlated with molecular information derived from clinical analytical procedures. When these archives are switched to clinical research, we need to establish a sufficient quality of the tissues for the type of molecular analysis to be performed, to gain the clinical information necessary for the research, such as follow-up data, and to pseudo-anonymize patients' personal information. The principal characteristics with which an archive starts to have the function of a biobank are the use of tissues for specific clinical research and pseudo-anonymization of the cases. Thus, pathology archives are clinical biorepositories that can take up the function of a biobank for specific case studies.

Because of the primary clinical orientation of pathology archives, participation in specific research must always be voluntary and collaborative from the pathologists that have the responsibility of the biorepository. This is because the clinical activity must be always maintained, with sufficient availability of tissues. Collaboration is requested for a careful choice of the tissue to be analyzed and, in case, for an accurate microdissection performed by the pathologist. The doctors of the original institution also have to be involved in the collection of clinical and follow-up information, to which they have free access because they are involved in the process of diagnostic/treatment process of the patients.

As already reported, privacy is highly guaranteed by the professional secrecy of the physicians involved, who have the duty to pseudo-anonymize the cases. The organization of the network can guarantee common rules and services especially if it is connected with a European infrastructure (BBMRI-ERIC).

Table 5.2 Basic principles for network organization

Box 2: How to organize the network?
The network is set up as a *virtual network* of pathology archives (samples + associated clinical data) for clinical research
Participation in the network and in the projects is voluntary and collaborative (these materials are residues from clinical procedures with specific requirements)
Clinical and follow-up information can be directly collected by pathologists because they also deal with the diagnostic procedures
Privacy is guaranteed by the professional secrecy of pathologists and other physicians that are directly involved in the diagnostic/treatment process, who have the duty to pseudo-anonymize the cases
The archives start to act as biobanks only in case of participation in a clinical research project and after the cases are pseudo-anonymized

5.7 Methodological Issues

Quality aspects are crucial for all tissue banks as the quality of the results of research absolutely depends on the quality of the material used for analyses [7]. Heterogeneity and variability of pre-analytical practices are a major source of error in analyzing biobanked specimens [8]. Pre-analytical phases of tissue processing have a deep impact on tissue quality. The first step in the process of tissue handling in the surgical theater is one of the most variable. The greatest contribution is given by the so-called warm ischemia time, which accounts for the time in which tissues remain in the body at 37 °C during the surgical procedures after the closure of the blood flow. This lapse of time could vary from minutes to hours and could account for data variability. The only possible solution to tackle the problem of the warm ischemia time is to document the ischemic time for the tissue samples (time from clamping of vascular supply or removal of sample to fixation) as part of the record of submission of the specimen to the pathology department and to the biorepositories [9, 10]. This phase is a common source of variability for biobanks of fresh frozen as well as fixed tissues biorepositories.

Among the pre-analytical variables associated with tissue harvesting and processing, transport from the surgical theater to the surgical-pathology laboratory could highly vary for duration (from hours to days) and type of transport and consequently could affect the recovery of higher quality biomolecules [11]. In the past, for clinical pathology biorepositories, transport from the surgical theater to the pathology department was mostly in formalin with a very variable time of a bad fixation process. Today's necessity is related to better standardization in the fixation process. Several possibilities are available for formalin-free transport of tissues, ranging from storage of tissues in ice to immersion of tissues in RNA later, or culture media [11], or transport under vacuum at 4 °C [12]. The latter is the best choice for a high level of preservation of macromolecules today.

During grossing of surgical samples, different tissue samples are obtained. In the case of tumor, for any of these specimens the location should be noted, reporting, e.g., if sampling was done at the border or at the center of the lesion. This aspect has major implications especially to study tumor heterogeneity.

The process of fixation encompasses three main variables: tissue thickness, volume of fixative, and time for fixation. Failure in optimizing these three aspects results in under- or over-fixation and suboptimal preservation of biomolecules [13]. A proper check of the abovementioned variables is mandatory for AT biobanking to achieve a better quality of both nucleic acids and protein. The optimal fixation time depends on the sample type and size. Usually, proper fixation time in formalin is considered between 12 and 24 h; clearly over-fixation with time exceeding 48 h results to be detrimental in RNA recovery [14]. To better preserve DNA and RNA, cold formalin fixation at 4 °C was also proposed [15].

Degradation of biomolecules does not end with the fixation step; tissue processing, paraffin embedding, and storage could also impact the recovery of biomolecules; therefore, for AT biobanking they should be optimized and the applied protocols should be documented. Tissue processing, encompassing clearing and paraffin impregnation, is fully automated, but not standardized. It could last from 4 to more than 12 h [10]. It is fundamental that tissues must be dehydrated, because residual water cannot be replaced by paraffin thus allowing further degradation. Improper tissue processing leads to inadequate replacement of water by paraffin and retaining of endogenous water in paraffin could cause further RNA hydrolysis and loss of protein antigenicity during storage [13, 16]. The use of low temperature melting paraffin is recommended for impregnation of tissues because it impacts on biomolecules recovery [10].

Even with optimal processing and storage conditions, like humidity and temperature, degradation of biomolecules is expected for FFPE tissue in long time archive storage [13, 17].

There are several alternatives to formalin fixation, in particular alcohol-based fixatives are reported to better preserve both nucleic acids and proteins. Among them are traditional alcohol fixatives, such as the modified Carnoy [18] or the BoonFix, a concentration of ethyl alcohol, PEG, and acetic acid [19]; commercial solutions such as the RCL-2® (Alphelys, Plaisir, France) [19] and PaxGene™ (Qiagen, Valencia, CA, USA) [20] as well as Umfix (Sakura Finetek USA, Inc., Torrance, CA, USA) [21] and FineFIX® (Milestone SrL, Bergamo, Italy) [18]. Among the proposed alternatives, traditional acetone fixation was coupled with the protective effect of HEPES-glutamic acid buffer in the commercial product called HOPE® (Polysciences, Inc., Warrington, PA, USA) [22]. The advantage of those fixatives resides in the better quality and quantity of recovered biomolecules in comparison to formalin. For RCL-2®, FineFix®, HOPE®, and PaxGene™ the possibility of performing proteomics analyses has been successfully investigated [11]. Regarding the use of those fixatives, there is only some skepticism about morphology and immunohistochemistry results [11]. Diagnostic use of these new fixatives is not suggested because different artifacts can be present in the fixation process. As a consequence, today's standardization, obtained with formalin and enabling comparison of histological and immunohistochemical results in any hospital of the world, could be lost. In AT biobanks one of those fixatives could be used to fix additional specimens for specific molecular analyses, such as proteomics.

From a methodological point of view, both extractive and in situ methods are possible in ATs. At large in situ methods, even if non-high throughput and usually non-quantitative, give the clear advantage of compartmentalizing the results in terms of tumor area (center, infiltrative border, histological differentiation, etc), of type of cells and intracellular level (nucleus, membrane, cytoplasm). This aspect is particularly advantageous for studying tumor heterogeneity. Mature in situ techniques are surely immunohistochemistry (IHC) and FISH. Nonetheless, even for IHC there are technical pitfalls in the analysis which could compromise correct interpretation of the analysis [23]. Nowadays, RNAscope®, employing a unique probe design strategy that allows target-specific signal amplification, has enabled single RNA molecule detection by in situ hybridization in FFPE specimens under standard bright-field microscopy [24].

Extractive methods are amenable in FFPE tissues both for nucleic acids and protein, preferably after a microdissection step to isolate the area of interest. Nucleic acids from AT are degraded and modified by adding methylol groups (CH_2-OH) to the nitrogenous bases. Those aspects are critical for extracting intact nucleic acids from FFPE. Different protocols and commercial solutions are available to extract nucleic acids from FFPE; they range from the use of digestion in a homemade or commercial solution, followed by phenol chloroform extraction or monophasic solutions to the use of commercial kits, which provide purification of the extracts, mainly by the use of spin columns and with magnetic tools [11]. There are no general recommendations to guide laboratories in their selection of protocols. Common steps in the extraction procedures are related to deparaffinization and proteolytic digestion. Extraction of nucleic acids from FFPE tissues requires an exhaustive proteolytic step to remove the protein crosslinking and allow solubilization of nucleic acids. In most cases proteolysis is achieved by proteinase K [11].

Several types of analyses are possible on nucleic acid extracts from FFPE material, ranging from PCR to high throughput methods (microarrays) and even whole sequencing. Usually, RNA analyses in FFPE are done after cDNA synthesis by reverse transcription. Although analysis of RNA isolated from FFPE tissues is widely used in biomedical research and molecular pathological diagnostics, it is important to point out that reverse transcription is the first and most confounding event in quantitative analysis in FFPE specimens because of its high variability both in protocol design and yield [25, 26].

Extraction of proteins from FFPE is possible both with in-house methods and commercial kits [27]. Protein extracts could be successfully submitted to western blot analyses as well as to reverse phase protein arrays [28, 29]. There are other "proteomic" approaches feasible in FFPE tissues [30], among them liquid-chromatography tandem mass spectrometry (LC-MS) has the advantage to be antibody free but demanding in terms of instrument requirements.

References

1. Council NR (2011) Toward precision medicine: building a knowledge network for biomedical research and a new taxonomy of disease. The National Academies Press, Washington, DC
2. Stanta G (2015) Tissue heterogeneity as a pre-analytical source of variability. In: Dietel M, Wittekind C, Bussolati G, von Winterfeld M (eds) Pre-analytics of pathological specimens in oncology, Recent results in cancer research, vol 199. Springer International Publishing, pp 35–43. https://doi.org/10.1007/978-3-319-13957-9_4
3. Stanta G, Zatloukal K, Riegman P (2014) White paper on retrospective studies in archive tissues. In: Paper presented at the tissue-based biomarkers for advancement of personalized Cancer treatment, Graz, Austria 28th–29th March, 2014. http://www.impactsnetwork.eu/userfiles/file/10WHITE%20PAPER25-09-14.pdf
4. BBMRI-ERIC: Biobanking and Biomolecular Resources Research Infrastructure. http://bbmri-eric.eu/
5. BBMRI-IT: Biobanking and Biomolecular Resources Research Infrastructure of Italy http://www.bbmri.it/nodo-bbmri.it

6. Rosai J (2011) Rosai and Ackerman's surgical pathology, 10th edn. Elsevier
7. Herpel E, Koleganova N, Schreiber B, Walter B, Kalle CV, Schirmacher P (2012) Structural requirements of research tissue banks derived from standardized project surveillance. Virchows Archiv 461(1):79–86. https://doi.org/10.1007/s00428-012-1258-3
8. Bevilacqua G, Bosman F, Dassesse T, Hofler H, Janin A, Langer R, Larsimont D, Morente MM, Riegman P, Schirmacher P, Stanta G, Zatloukal K, Caboux E, Hainaut P (2010) The role of the pathologist in tissue banking: European consensus expert group report. Virchows Archiv 456(4):449–454. https://doi.org/10.1007/s00428-010-0887-7
9. Bray SE, Paulin FE, Fong SC, Baker L, Carey FA, Levison DA, Steele RJ, Kernohan NM (2010) Gene expression in colorectal neoplasia: modifications induced by tissue ischaemic time and tissue handling protocol. Histopathology 56(2):240–250. https://doi.org/10.1111/j.1365-2559.2009.03470.x
10. Hewitt SM, Lewis FA, Cao Y, Conrad RC, Cronin M, Danenberg KD, Goralski TJ, Langmore JP, Raja RG, Williams PM, Palma JF, Warrington JA (2008) Tissue handling and specimen preparation in surgical pathology: issues concerning the recovery of nucleic acids from formalin-fixed, paraffin-embedded tissue. Arch Pathol Lab Med 132(12):1929–1935. https://doi.org/10.1043/1543-2165-132.12.1929
11. Bonin S, Stanta G (2013) Nucleic acid extraction methods from fixed and paraffin-embedded tissues in cancer diagnostics. Expert Rev Mol Diagn 13(3):271–282. https://doi.org/10.1586/erm.13.14
12. Bussolati G, Chiusa L, Cimino A, D'Armento G (2008) Tissue transfer to pathology labs: under vacuum is the safe alternative to formalin. Virchows Archiv 452(2):229–231. https://doi.org/10.1007/s00428-007-0529-x
13. Xie R, Chung JY, Ylaya K, Williams RL, Guerrero N, Nakatsuka N, Badie C, Hewitt SM (2011) Factors influencing the degradation of archival formalin-fixed paraffin-embedded tissue sections. J Histochem Cytochem 59(4):356–365. https://doi.org/10.1369/0022155411398488
14. Chung JY, Braunschweig T, Hewitt SM (2006) Optimization of recovery of RNA from formalin-fixed, paraffin-embedded tissue. Diagn Mol Pathol 15(4):229–236. https://doi.org/10.1097/01.pdm.0000213468.91139.2d
15. Bussolati G, Annaratone L, Medico E, D'Armento G, Sapino A (2011) Formalin fixation at low temperature better preserves nucleic acid integrity. PLoS One 6(6):e21043. https://doi.org/10.1371/journal.pone.0021043
16. Chung JY, Braunschweig T, Williams R, Guerrero N, Hoffmann KM, Kwon M, Song YK, Libutti SK, Hewitt SM (2008) Factors in tissue handling and processing that impact RNA obtained from formalin-fixed, paraffin-embedded tissue. J Histochem Cytochem 56(11):1033–1042. https://doi.org/10.1369/jhc.2008.951863
17. von Ahlfen S, Missel A, Bendrat K, Schlumpberger M (2007) Determinants of RNA quality from FFPE samples. PLoS One 2(12):e1261. https://doi.org/10.1371/journal.pone.0001261
18. Dotti I, Bonin S, Basili G, Nardon E, Balani A, Siracusano S, Zanconati F, Palmisano S, De Manzini N, Stanta G (2010) Effects of formalin, methacarn, and fineFIX fixatives on RNA preservation. Diagn Mol Pathol 19(2):112–122
19. van Essen HF, Verdaasdonk MA, Elshof SM, de Weger RA, van Diest PJ (2010) Alcohol based tissue fixation as an alternative for formaldehyde: influence on immunohistochemistry. J Clin Pathol 63(12):1090–1094. https://doi.org/10.1136/jcp.2010.079905
20. Nietner T, Jarutat T, Mertens A (2012) Systematic comparison of tissue fixation with alternative fixatives to conventional tissue fixation with buffered formalin in a xenograft-based model. Virchows Archiv 461(3):259–269. https://doi.org/10.1007/s00428-012-1248-5
21. Nassiri M, Ramos S, Zohourian H, Vincek V, Morales AR, Nadji M (2008) Preservation of biomolecules in breast cancer tissue by a formalin-free histology system. BMC Clin Pathol 8:1. https://doi.org/10.1186/1472-6890-8-1
22. Kahler D, Alexander C, Schultz H, Abdullah M, Branscheid D, Lindner B, Zabel P, Vollmer E, Goldmann T (2010) Proteomics out of the archive: two-dimensional electrophoresis and

mass spectrometry using HOPE-fixed, paraffin-embedded tissues. J Histochem Cytochem 58(3):221–228. https://doi.org/10.1369/jhc.2009.954065
23. Bussolati G, Leonardo E (2008) Technical pitfalls potentially affecting diagnoses in immunohistochemistry. J Clin Pathol 61(11):1184–1192. https://doi.org/10.1136/jcp.2007.047720
24. Wang H, Su N, Wang LC, Wu X, Bui S, Nielsen A, Vo HT, Luo Y, Ma XJ (2014) Quantitative ultrasensitive bright-field RNA in situ hybridization with RNAscope. Methods Mol Biol 1211:201–212. https://doi.org/10.1007/978-1-4939-1459-3_16
25. Kashofer K, Viertler C, Pichler M, Zatloukal K (2013) Quality control of RNA preservation and extraction from paraffin-embedded tissue: implications for RT-PCR and microarray analysis. PLoS One 8(7):e70714. https://doi.org/10.1371/journal.pone.0070714
26. Nardon E, Donada M, Bonin S, Dotti I, Stanta G (2009) Higher random oligo concentration improves reverse transcription yield of cDNA from bioptic tissues and quantitative RT-PCR reliability. Exp Mol Pathol 87(2):146–151
27. Nirmalan NJ, Harnden P, Selby PJ, Banks RE (2009) Development and validation of a novel protein extraction methodology for quantitation of protein expression in formalin-fixed paraffin-embedded tissues using western blotting. J Pathol 217(4):497–506. https://doi.org/10.1002/path.2504
28. Malinowsky K, Wolff C, Ergin B, Berg D, Becker KF (2010) Deciphering signaling pathways in clinical tissues for personalized medicine using protein microarrays. J Cell Physiol 225(2):364–370. https://doi.org/10.1002/jcp.22307
29. Shi SR, Taylor CR, Fowler CB, Mason JT (2013) Complete solubilization of formalin-fixed, paraffin-embedded tissue may improve proteomic studies. Proteomics Clin Appl 7(3–4):264–272. https://doi.org/10.1002/prca.201200031
30. Fowler CB, O'Leary TJ, Mason JT (2013) Toward improving the proteomic analysis of formalin-fixed, paraffin-embedded tissue. Expert Rev Proteomics 10(4):389–400. https://doi.org/10.1586/14789450.2013.820531

Chapter 6
Biobanking Best Practices and Publication Standards

Jim Vaught

Abstract Initially focused primarily on collecting samples for diagnostic purposes in pathology settings, biobanks have evolved into complex organizations engaged in advancing personalized medicine and translational research. This evolution has involved the development of biobanking best practices and the transformation of a field driven by empirical approaches into the emerging area of biospecimen science. It has become increasingly important to develop evidence-based practices for collecting specimens and data which can be shared with confidence with international collaborators. Aside from these technical approaches, other factors play crucial roles, such as developing publication standards; ethical and regulatory issues; business planning and sustainability; and approaches to data collection and sharing.

Keywords Biobanking · Best practices · Publication standards · Biospecimen

6.1 Introduction

Biobanking is often thought of as the simple technical and logistical approaches to collecting, processing, and storing biospecimens ("biospecimens" as used in this chapter includes liquid samples such as blood, urine, saliva, as well as tissue and cellular samples). However, biobanking is a more complex endeavor and is the term which incorporates the physical infrastructure used to house specimens and data systems, as well as the policies and procedures which are developed to govern its operations. And usually one thinks of large warehouses of freezers with frozen blood or tissue samples, or pathology departments with collections of formalin-fixed, paraffin-embedded (FFPE) tissues. Generally, these pathology collections were the most prevalent in the origins of biobanks over 100 years ago [1]. These collections, generally of the FFPE type, were (and still are) necessary for patient diagnoses in clinical centers. Biobanking grew out of the recognition that such collections can also contribute significantly to biomedical research endeavors. Over the

J. Vaught (✉)
International Prevention Research Institute, Kensington, MD, USA

P. Hainaut et al. (eds.), *Biobanking of Human Biospecimens*,
https://doi.org/10.1007/978-3-030-55901-4_6

decades the value of pathology collections to research led to more organized efforts to leverage such diagnostic specimen collections into translational research programs. Biobanking is now considered a cornerstone in the development of personalized (or precision) medicine [2]. The diversity of specimen types collected for such studies has expanded to a variety of tissue, liquid, and cellular samples procured and processed in multiple formats. Some high-profile biobanking failures, and the general sense that biospecimen quality was not adequately controlled, led to the development of best practices, the evolution of biospecimen methods research [3], and generally the recognition that biobanking needed to "come of age" and become a "science" in its own right [4, 5].

In this chapter, the development of biobanking best practices will be discussed, along with the roles of publication standards, and certification and accreditation standards based on best practices.

6.2 Biobanking Best Practices

6.2.1 The Evolution of Biobanking Best Practices

As biobanks became larger and more complex in terms of the numbers and types of specimens and data comprising the collections, a series of high-profile best practices were published. The International Society for Biological and Environmental Repositories (ISBER) published the first edition of its best practices in 2005, followed by three new editions, the latest published in 2018 [6]. Other best practices have been published by the US National Cancer Institute (NCI) [7], International Agency for Research on Cancer (IARC), and the Organisation for Economic Cooperation and Development (OECD). Several reviews have outlined the development of multiple international best practice documents [8, 9]. Generally, biobanking best practices contain documented procedures developed empirically by the larger institutional and commercial biobanks such as shown in Fig. 6.1, which tend to have well-developed quality management, information systems, and specimen handling processes in place. As biobanking has developed into biospecimen science, there has been a trend toward developing evidence-based standard procedures for incorporation into best practices. Engel et al. discuss the NCI's approach to developing such procedures and provide a detailed example for snap freezing of postsurgical tissue specimens [10].

The following shows the major contents headings from the NCI *Best Practices for Biospecimen Resources* [7]:

(a) **Scope, Applicability, and Implementation.**
(b) **Technical and Operational Best Practices**

1. Biospecimen resource management and operations
2. Biospecimen collection, processing, storage, retrieval, and dissemination

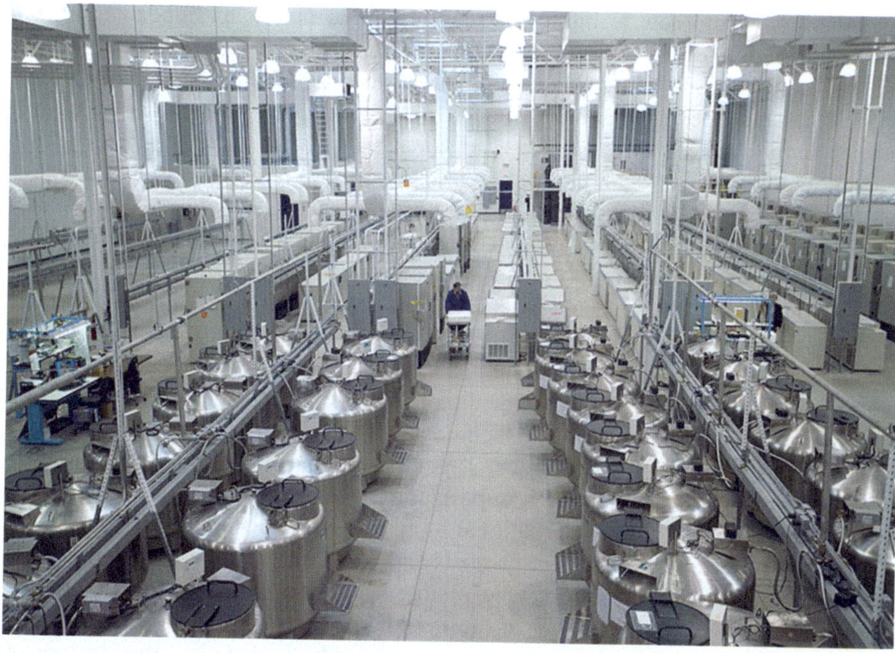

Fig. 6.1 US National Cancer Institute Biobank with liquid nitrogen and mechanical freezers. (Photo courtesy of Leidos Biomedical Research, Incorporated)

3. Quality management
4. Biosafety
5. Collecting and managing clinical data
6. Biospecimen resource informatics: data management and inventory control and tracking

(c) **Ethical, Legal, and Policy Best Practices**

1. Principles for responsible custodianship
2. Informed consent
3. Privacy and confidentiality protections
4. Access to biospecimens and data
5. Intellectual property and resource sharing
6. Conflicts of interest

Generally, the technical and operational practices for biobanks have developed to a point where most operations follow similar or identical procedures. Current best practices documents and other publications provide detailed recommendations concerning the standard methods for collection, processing, storage, and shipping of blood, tissue, urine, saliva, and other commonly collected specimens [11–13]. Epidemiologic studies may involve a complex array of sample collections requiring the development of multiple standard operating procedures (SOPs) [14]. Emerging specimen types and new technologies require regular review and updates to standard practices. As discussed in the section Toward Evidence-Based Practices, there are still many unresolved questions concerning the optimal methods for collecting, processing, and storing specimens, due to the effects of pre-analytical variables and other potential biases.

In terms of ethical, legal, and policy practices, those tend to be more unsettled and controversial (see Section Ethical, Legal, and Social Issues). In addition, such issues are more subject to local and national regulations, making international collaborations more difficult in terms of the exchange of specimens and data [15].

With the proliferation of best practices from a variety of sources, as well as the increasing number and complexity of biobanks, it has become important to ask whether there should be one overarching set of best practices which can be adopted internationally. A review of international biobanking best practices in 2010 listed 14 organizations which had published such documents at that time [16], making for a confusing array of recommendations. This situation is difficult to resolve for the reasons discussed above, making it important to develop and adopt evidence-based practices. ISBER and other international biobanking organizations are engaged in attempting to educate biobanking scientists and move the field toward international coordination and harmonization. One of the more comprehensive efforts, and a good model for the future, is that of the Biobanking and Biomolecular Resources Research Infrastructure (BBMRI), organized and funded by the European Commission [17], which is coordinating efforts in Europe and elsewhere to develop sustainable biobanking programs. BBMRI's initiatives include hosting and participating in biobanking-related workshops and training programs, and developing educational materials which will hopefully result in more international cooperation and coordination [17, 18].

6.3 Evidence-Based Practices and Standards

6.3.1 Specimen Quality Issues

As biospecimen science has developed over the past 10 years its practitioners have learned valuable lessons from some high-profile failures in studies, at least partially due to biospecimen handling and quality issues. As noted by Spruessel et al. [19] in their study of the effects of tissue ischemia duration on gene expression: "While scientists control variables in their experimental settings and try to minimize them as much as possible, they usually barely know about the background of clinical samples."

In the NIH project The Cancer Genome Atlas [20], there were some early specimen quality failures due to retrospective tumor samples procured from existing frozen collections not meeting the pathology or molecular quality standards set for the study [21]. More than half the specimens initially collected for the project failed quality control. Ultimately the project leadership decided to transition from retrospective specimen collection to prospective collection using carefully controlled standard protocols. This approach led to a quality success rate of over 80%.

In establishing the treatment protocol for potential breast cancer patients, HER2 (human epidermal growth factor 2) assays are performed [22] in order to assess whether treatment with Herceptin will be effective. In 2007, the College of American Pathologists (CAP) [23] and the American Society for Clinical Oncology (ASCO) [24] completed a study of the interlaboratory variability of HER2 assays in a number of clinical laboratories. The study determined that the rates of false positives and false negatives approached 20%. In publishing their findings and recommendations [25, 26] ASCO and CAP reported that at least some of the issues with the HER2 assays originated with variability in the breast specimen fixation methods.

Many other examples of the effects of pre-analytical variables on specimen quality and variability have been published, although as discussed in the following sections, efforts to compile a comprehensive literature concerning biospecimen science are fairly recent developments. For examples of such studies, see papers by Koury et al. [27], "Delay to formalin fixation effect on breast biomarkers" and Hewitt et al. [28], "Impact of preanalytic factors on the design and application of integral biomarkers for directing patient therapy." Poste [29], in "Biospecimens, biomarkers, and burgeoning data: the imperative for more rigorous research standards," emphasizes the importance of developing approaches to mitigate the effects of biospecimen pre-analytical variables. Ransohoff and Gourlay [30] discuss the sources of bias in biomarker studies, which can involve the effects of specimen handling. In addition to the pre-analytical variables, such effects can include batch effects in analyzing samples and differences in the sources of samples, for example, among cases and controls (Table 6.1).

6.3.2 Quality Management Systems

As biobanking best practices have developed, and biospecimen science has emerged in the wake of the issues discussed in the last section, the development of quality management systems (QMS) has become a major focus in the "professionalization" of biobanks. In general terms, biobanks have adopted the quality assurance (QA) and quality control (QC) practices long utilized in clinical chemistry laboratories, with additional practices developed which are unique to biobanks [31, 32].

Basic QMS for biobanks requires SOPs for each function of the operation [33–36]. Staff should be trained in the SOPs and procedures should be in place for periodic review, and an electronic document control system should be in place. The basics of quality management are described in detail in the current major best practices editions from ISBER, NCI, OECD, and other organizations [16].

As biobanking and biospecimen science have evolved, so have quality management systems. The early adopters of more comprehensive QMS were biobanks which collected and stored biospecimens for clinical applications and were subject

Table 6.1 Adapted from Ransohoff and Gourlay, J. Clin Oncol 2010 [30]

Source of bias	Location of bias: before or after specimens are received in the laboratory Before After	Example
Features of subjects, Determined in selection: Age Sex Comorbid conditions Medications	X	Cancer subjects are male, whereas control subjects are mainly female Bias: Assay results may depend on sex
Specimen collection	X	Cancer specimens come from one clinic, whereas control specimens come from a different clinic Bias: Assay results may depend on conditions that differ between clinics
Specimen storage and handling	X X	Cancer specimens are stored for 10 years because it takes longer to collect them, whereas control specimens are collected and stored over 1 year Bias: Assay results may vary with duration of storage, or with different numbers of thaw-freeze cycles
Specimen analysis	X	Cancer specimens are run on 1 day, whereas control specimens are run on a different day Bias: Assay results may depend on day of analysis in a machine that "wanders" over time

Note: The table shows examples of different sources of bias and the location of the bias before or after specimens are received in the laboratory. The list is not exhaustive; other biases may be important, and the biases listed may or may not be important in any given research study, depending on details of biology and technology (i.e., what is being measured and how it might be influenced)

to FDA inspection. These operations developed QMS based on Good Manufacturing Practices (cGMP) [37]. cGMP involves adhering to strict standards in terms of SOPs; security; detailed documentation of equipment installation; performance and maintenance; IT systems; and a thoroughly documented chain of custody for all samples and reagents. More recently some biobanks, in particular those which engage in international collaborations, have undergone the certification process of the International Organization for Standardization (ISO) [38]. The ISO standard which is generally adopted for biobanks is ISO 9001 [39]. However, ISO 9001 was developed for general quality management purposes, and not specifically for biobanking operations. A more biobank-specific ISO standard (ISO 20387) was developed by an international committee with experts from ISBER and other organizations and published in 2018 [40]. Any ISO certification process is comprehensive and successful completion of the application provides assurance that the organization is committed to meeting high-quality management standards.

6.3.3 Evidence-Based Methods

Although the recognition of the role of quality management was an important development in biobanking, issues concerning uneven quality of biospecimens remain a major obstacle to the generation of reliable analytical results [21]. Through a number of challenges due to specimen quality issues, as described above, the development of evidence-based procedures has become a priority for many biobanks. The ISBER Best Practices recommend pilot studies to optimize specimen collection and processing procedures [6]. However, often such biospecimen methodology studies are developed only for local biobank or laboratory use and are not widely disseminated or published [4, 5, 41]. The approach which should be taken to develop a new biobanking effort is exemplified by the UK Biobank [42, 43]. In 2008, the project leadership published a series of articles in the *International Journal of Epidemiology* which detailed the preliminary methods studies performed to establish the optimal approaches to collecting specimens for the project, which ultimately included 500,000 participants. The methods studies included assessments of the stability of blood and analytes, automated sample processing, and a novel automated blood fractionation system [44].

Starting in 2008 organizations such as the US NCI Biospecimen Research Network [45] and SPIDIA (Standardization and improvement of generic pre-analytical tools and procedures for in vitro diagnostics [46]) began to take a more organized approach to study the effects of pre-analytical variables and other factors on the quality of specimens and the reliability of downstream analyses [45, 47]. Depending on the analyses to be performed pre-analytical variables may include freeze-thaw cycles for frozen specimens, time intervals from sample collection to stabilization, drugs taken by surgical patients, and other factors [19].

Both the BRN and SPIDIA have published results of their studies [48, 49]. In addition, the NCI maintains the Biospecimen Research Database (BRD) [45], which is a compilation of summaries and conclusions from over 2000 biospecimen research papers from dozens of journals. Figure 6.2 shows the BRD's approach to searching for papers according to the stage of the "biospecimen life cycle," integrated with examples of potential pre-analytical variables which may affect specimen quality and analytical results.

Since biospecimen science involves multiple scientific disciplines, such publications are found in clinical chemistry, pathology, epidemiology, genomics, proteomics, and many other journals devoted to basic, translational and clinical research. NCI investigators from the Biorepository and Biospecimen Research Branch (BBRB) have published reviews on topics extracted from BRD papers [10] as an approach to expand the literature on evidence-based biobanking practices. An example of a paper concerning how pre-analytical variables can affect urine

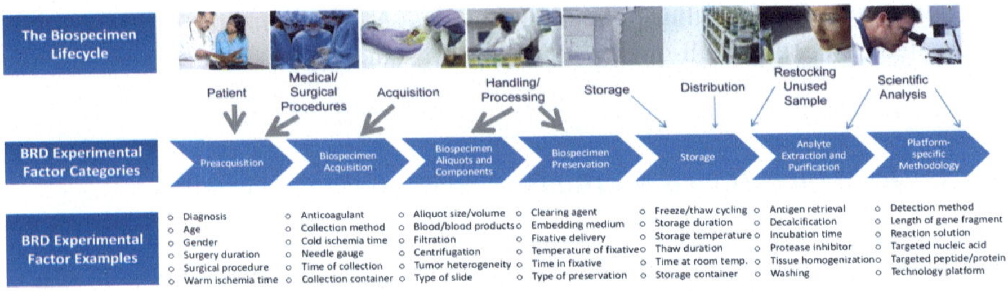

Fig. 6.2 The NCI Biospecimen Research Database search categories, showing stages of specimen acquisition, processing and storage, and potential pre-analytical variables (factors)

collected for metabolomics studies, curated and summarized in the BRD, is shown in Fig. 6.3. However, the literature concerning the effects of pre-analytical variables and other factors which may affect specimen quality is often conflicting. Additional comprehensive efforts will be needed to arrive at evidence-based standards which are widely adopted in the basic and clinical research settings. The conflicting data in the literature and economic factors continue to be obstacles to the adoption of new biospecimen collection and processing standards.

6.3.4 Publication Standards

Another issue which is an obstacle to the development of evidence-based biobanking standard procedures is the general lack of rigor in reporting specimen collection, processing and storage conditions, and other sample handling details in manuscripts. This issue is made even more difficult to resolve due to the multiple scientific disciplines which are involved in biospecimen-related research. As already noted, articles from studies which involve significant collection and use of specimens may appear in journals which focus on pathology, epidemiology, genomics, proteomics, clinical chemistry, and other areas of research. During the past 10 years, several sets of standards have been published which encourage publishers, authors, editors, and reviewers of manuscripts to ensure inclusion of sufficient details about specimen collection and handling, in order for the validity of the results to be evaluated. The REMARK guidelines [50, 51] were developed primarily to guide investigators in reporting standards for biomarker discovery and development but included several recommendations concerning specimen handling. More recently, an international committee of experts led by the NCI BBRB, developed Biospecimen Reporting for Improved Study Quality (BRISQ) [52, 53]. BRISQ is a set of standards which is designed to encourage authors to include a standard list of specimen variables in their manuscripts' materials and methods. BRISQ variables are organized into three Tiers according to a set of priorities and consideration of the complexity of collection of the information. BRISQ Tier 1 includes the items which are most important to report and should be readily available to investigators, such as

Standard operating procedures for pre-analytical handling of blood and urine for metabolomic studies and biobanks.

Author(s): Bernini P, Bertini I, Luchinat C, Nincheri P, Staderini S, Turano P

Publication: *J Biomol NMR*, 2011, Vol. 49, Page 231-43

PubMed

Found in 1 study(s)

Study Purpose:

The purpose of this study was to determine the effects of centrifugation speed (450 x g, 1000 x g, 3000 x g, or 11000 x g), filtering or adding sodium azide to centrifuged or uncentrifuged specimens, frozen storage temperature, and storage of preserved or unpreserved specimens at -80 degrees C and subsequently at room temperature on NMR profiles. Urine from 2 individuals was aliquoted, centrifuged for 5 min at 4 degrees C or left uncentrifuged, subjected to various pretreatments (filtration, enzymatic inhibitors, sodium azide or none), frozen for 1 week or used fresh, and stored for up to 24 h at room temperature.

Specimens: Fluid - Urine ***Preservation Types:*** Frozen, Other Preservative, None (Fresh) ***Diagnoses:*** Not specified

Platforms:

Small molecule - NMR

Carbohydrate - NMR

Summary of Findings:

The difference between the first component of the spectra from the centrifuged and uncentrifuged specimens was greatest when the centrifugation speed was 1,000 or 3,000 relative centrifugal force (RCF). NMR spectra from specimens centrifuged at 11,000 RCF were closer to those in the specimens that were uncentrifuged, which the authors attribute to breaking down of the cells. The effect of centrifugation speeds was more pronounced in urine with a high cellular content. When urine was centrifuged prior to frozen storage for a week, the NMR profile was different from that when specimens were not centrifuged prior to frozen storage, but the magnitude of the difference was greater when the specimens were stored at -80 degrees C rather than in liquid nitrogen (8% as much change) or when NMR profiles from fresh centrifuged and uncentrifuged urine were compared (9% as much change). Importantly, changes observed after freezing or centrifugation were very small compared to the interindividual variability. Fresh or previously frozen, but unpreserved urine stored for 24 h at room temperature showed a spectral shift in pH sensitive metabolites as the specimen became more alkaline. Importantly, with storage at room temperature, succinate and acetate increased while urea, lactate, and glutamate decreased. However, specimens that were centrifuged and filtered showed fewer changes in spectra with storage at room temperature than specimens that were preserved with sodium azide, those that were unpreserved, or those only centrifuged prior to analysis or storage at -80 degrees C. When urine was stored for 24 h in an inert atmosphere rather than the normal atmosphere, the only difference was a slight reduction in the change in succinate. Addition of acetohydroxamic acid inhibited the decrease in urea with storage, and addition of EDTA at least partially attenuated the change in succinate and urea with storage.

Fig. 6.3 Example of a paper curated and summarized in the NCI Biospecimen Research Database. (From [45])

sample type; collection method; stabilization method; storage temperature and duration; shipping temperature. Tier 2 includes items which may be important pre-analytical variables for some analyses and should be reported if available, such as time intervals between collection and stabilization of the specimens, and time the samples remain in fixative. Tier 3 includes items which may be less commonly recorded such as the number of times a sample has been thawed and refrozen; details of sample shipping; time from cessation of blood flow to biospecimen excision (warm ischemic time). Both REMARK and BRISQ were published simultaneously in several journals, and their implementation has been endorsed by multiple journals.

A newer specimen collection documentation scheme is the **S**tandard **PRE**-analytical **C**ode (SPREC) [54–56], which involves applying a standard set of codes to a specimen collection procedure. An example is (quoting from [56]):

> Solid tissue or cytologic specimen **TIS-BPS-N-B-RNL-A-A**. This corresponds to a solid tissue (TIS) specimen that has been collected as a biopsy (BPS), with no warm ischemia (N), with cold ischemia of <10 min (B), fixed in RNALater (RNL) for <15 min (A) and stored in a 0.5- to 2 mL polypropylene tube at a temperature between −85 and −60 °C (A). Biopsies, obtained either at time of traditional surgery, laparoscopy, or puncture, and cytologic specimens such as fine needle aspirates, are assigned the same SPREC.

All of these initiatives concerning quality management, biospecimen methodology research, the development of evidence-based practices, and reporting standards are significant advances in biobanking. However, such initiatives will only be effective if evidence-based standards are incorporated into biobanking best practices and widely adopted. That has yet to happen.

6.4 Conclusion

Biobanks have evolved from collections of specimens where collection, processing, and storage were not well-controlled into a branch of science for which there are professional organizations, best practices, and international collaborations involving complex logistics and regulations.

The empirical biobanking practices of the past are giving way to careful consideration of pre-analytical variables which affect specimen quality, and the development of evidence-based practices.

Quality management systems and more highly trained technical staff have led to the "professionalization" of biobanking. Recognition of the importance of publishing biospecimen science articles has led to the development of multiple reporting guidelines such as BRISQ and SPREC.

References

1. Eiseman EHS (1999) Handbook of human tissue sources: a national resource of human tissue samples. RAND Corporation, Santa Monica, CA
2. Collins FS, Varmus H (2015) A new initiative on precision medicine. N Engl J Med 372(9):793–795
3. Moore HM, Compton CC, Alper J, Vaught JB (2011) International approaches to advancing biospecimen science. Cancer Epidemiol Biomarker Prev 20:729–732
4. Vaught JB (2006) Biorepository and biospecimen science: a new focus for CEBP. Cancer Epidemiol Biomarker Prev 15:1572–1573
5. Vaught JB, Henderson MK, Compton CC (2012) Biospecimens and biorepositories: from afterthought to science. Cancer Epidemiol Biomarker Prev 21:253–255

6. Campbell L, Astrin J, DeSouza Y, Giri J, Patel A et al (2018) The 2018 revision of the ISBER best practices: summary of changes and the editorial team's development process. Biopreserv Biobank 16:3–6. https://doi.org/10.1089/bio.2018.0001
7. NCI best practices for biospecimen resources. http://biospecimens.cancer.gov/bestpractices/. Accessed 15 Feb 2021
8. Vaught J, Lockhart NC (2012) The evolution of biobanking best practices. Clin Chim Acta 413:1569–1575
9. Vaught J, Kelly A, Hewitt R (2009) A review of international biobanks and networks: success factors and key benchmarks. Biopreserv Biobank 7:143–150
10. Engel KB, Vaught J, Moore HM (2014) National Cancer Institute biospecimen evidence-based practices: a novel approach to pre-analytical standardization. Biopreserv Biobank 12:148–150
11. Garcia-Closas M, Moore LE, Rabkin CS, Franklin T, Struewing J et al (2006) Quantitation of DNA in buccal cell samples collected in epidemiological studies. Biomarkers 11:472–479
12. Jewell SD, Srinivasan M, McCart LM, Williams N, Grizzle WH et al (2002) Analysis of the molecular quality of human tissues: an experience from the cooperative human tissue network. Am J Clin Pathol 118:733–741
13. Vaught JB (2006) Blood collection, shipment, processing, and storage. Cancer Epidemiol Biomarker Prev 15:1582–1584
14. Cortes B, Schiffman M, Herrero R, Hildesheim A, Jimenez S et al (2010) Establishment and operation of a biorepository for molecular epidemiologic studies in Costa Rica. Cancer Epidemiol Biomarker Prev 19:916–922
15. Vaught J, Bledsoe M, Watson P (2014) Biobanking on multiple continents: will international coordination follow? Biopreserv Biobank 12:1–2
16. Vaught JB, Caboux E, Hainaut P (2010) International efforts to develop biospecimen best practices. Cancer Epidemiol Biomarker Prev 19:912–915
17. van Ommen GJ, Tornwall O, Brechot C, Dagher G, Galli J, et al 2014 BBMRI-ERIC as a resource for pharmaceutical and life science industries: the development of biobank-based expert centres. Eur J Human Genet
18. Viertler C, Zatloukal K (2008) [Biobanking and biomolecular resources research infrastructure (BBMRI). Implications for pathology]. Der Pathologe 29 Suppl 2:210–3
19. Spruessel A, Steimann G, Jung M, Lee SA, Carr T et al (2004) Tissue ischemia time affects gene and protein expression patterns within minutes following surgical tumor excision. BioTechniques 36:1030–1037
20. The cancer genome atlas. http://cancergenome.nih.gov/. Accessed 15 Feb 2021
21. Compton C (2007) Getting to personalized cancer medicine: taking out the garbage. Cancer 110:1641–1643
22. Perez EA, Press MF, Dueck AC, Jenkins RB, Kim C et al (2013) Immunohistochemistry and fluorescence in situ hybridization assessment of HER2 in clinical trials of adjuvant therapy for breast cancer (NCCTG N9831, BCIRG 006, and BCIRG 005). Breast Cancer Res Treat 138:99–108
23. College of American Pathologists. http://www.cap.org/. Accessed 15 Feb 2021
24. American Society of Clinical Oncology. http://www.asco.org/. Accessed 15 Feb 2021
25. Wolff AC, Hammond ME, Schwartz JN, Hagerty KL, Allred DC et al (2007) American Society of Clinical Oncology/College of American Pathologists guideline recommendations for human epidermal growth factor receptor 2 testing in breast cancer. Arch Pathol Lab Med 131:18–43
26. Wolff AC, Hammond ME, Hicks DG, Dowsett M, McShane LM et al (2013) Recommendations for human epidermal growth factor receptor 2 testing in breast cancer: American Society of Clinical Oncology/College of American Pathologists clinical practice guideline update. J Clin Oncol 31:3997–4013
27. Khoury T, Sait S, Hwang H, Chandrasekhar R, Wilding G et al (2009) Delay to formalin fixation effect on breast biomarkers. Mod Pathol 22:1457–1467
28. Hewitt SM, Badve SS, True LD (2012) Impact of preanalytic factors on the design and application of integral biomarkers for directing patient therapy. Clin Cancer Res 18:1524–1530

29. Poste G (2012) Biospecimens, biomarkers, and burgeoning data: the imperative for more rigorous research standards. Trends Mol Med 18:717–722
30. Ransohoff DF, Gourlay ML (2010) Sources of bias in specimens for research about molecular markers for cancer. J Clin Oncol 28:698–704
31. Betsou F, Barnes R, Burke T, Coppola D, Desouza Y et al (2009) Human biospecimen research: experimental protocol and quality control tools. Cancer Epidemiol Biomarker Prev 18:1017–1025
32. Betsou F, Gunter E, Clements J, DeSouza Y, Goddard KA et al (2013) Identification of evidence-based biospecimen quality-control tools: a report of the International Society for Biological and Environmental Repositories (ISBER) biospecimen science working group. J Mol Diagn 15:3–16
33. Carter A, Betsou F (2011) Quality assurance in cancer biobanking. Biopreserv Biobank 9:157–163
34. Carter A, Betsou F, Clark BJ (2011) Quality management and accreditation of research tissue banks. Virchows Arch 458:247–248; author reply 9–50
35. Chaigneau C, Cabioch T, Beaumont K, Betsou F (2007) Serum biobank certification and the establishment of quality controls for biological fluids: examples of serum biomarker stability after temperature variation. Clin Chem Lab Med 45:1390–1395
36. Vaught JA, Peakman T et al (2014) Critical issues in international biobanking. Clin Chem 60:1368–1374
37. FDA current good manufacturing processes. http://www.fda.gov/Drugs/DevelopmentApprovalProcess/Manufacturing/ucm169105.htm. Accessed 15 Feb 2021
38. International Organization for Standardization (ISO). http://www.iso.org/iso/home.html. Accessed 15 Feb 2021
39. International Organization of Standards: 9001 Quality Management. http://www.iso.org/iso/iso_9000. Accessed 15 Feb 2021
40. International Organization of Standardization ISO 20387:2018. Biotechnology—biobanking—general requirements for biobanking: https://www.iso.org/standard/67888.html. Accessed 15 Feb 2021
41. Vaught JB, Hsing AW (2010) Methodologic data: important foundation for molecular and biomarker studies. Cancer Epidemiol Biomarker Prev 19:901–902
42. Peakman TC, Elliott P (2008) The UK biobank sample handling and storage validation studies. Int J Epidemiol 37(Suppl 1):i2–i6
43. UK biobank home page. http://www.ukbiobank.ac.uk/. Accessed 15 Feb 2021
44. The UK biobank sample handling and storage validation studies. http://ije.oxfordjournals.org/content/37/suppl_1.toc. Accessed 15 Feb 2021
45. NCI Biospecimen Research Network. https://biospecimens.cancer.gov/about/researchnetwork/default.asp. Accessed 15 Feb 2021
46. Standardisation and improvement of generic pre-analytical tools and procedures for in-vitro diagnostics (SPIDIA). http://www.spidia.eu/. Accessed 15 Feb 2021
47. Moore HM, Compton CC, Lim MD et al (2009) Biospecimen research network symposium: advancing cancer research through biospecimen science. Cancer Res 69:6770–6772
48. SPIDIA research publications. http://www.spidia.eu/publications/articles/. Accessed 15 Feb 2021
49. NCI Biospecimen Research Network publications. https://biospecimens.cancer.gov/about/sp.asp
50. Altman DG, McShane LM, Sauerbrei W, Taube SE (2012) Reporting recommendations for tumor marker prognostic studies (REMARK): explanation and elaboration. PLoS Med 9:e1001216
51. McShane LM, Altman DG, Sauerbrei W, Taube SE, Gion M et al (2005) REporting recommendations for tumour MARKer prognostic studies (REMARK). Eur J Cancer 41:1690–1696
52. Moore HM, Kelly AB, Jewell SD, McShane LM, Clark DP et al (2011) Biospecimen reporting for improved study quality (BRISQ). Cancer Cytopathol 119:92–101

53. Moore HM, Kelly A, McShane LM, Vaught J (2012) Biospecimen reporting for improved study quality (BRISQ). Clin Chim Acta 413:1305
54. Nanni U, Betsou F, Riondino S, Rossetti L, Spila A et al (2012) SPRECware: software tools for standard PREanalytical code (SPREC) labeling - effective exchange and search of stored biospecimens. Int J Biol Markers 27:e272–e279
55. Nussbeck SY, Benson EE, Betsou F, Guadagni F, Lehmann S, Umbach N (2013) Is there a protocol for using the SPREC? Biopreserv Biobank 11:260–266
56. Betsou F, Lehmann S, Ashton G, Barnes M, Benson EE et al (2010) Standard preanalytical coding for biospecimens: defining the sample PREanalytical code. Cancer Epidemiol Biomarker Prev 19:1004–1011

Chapter 7
Ethical Challenges for Biobanks: Two Sides of the Coin

Kirsi Vähäkangas, Suchetana De, and Pierre Hainaut

Abstract The many ethical challenges in biobanking include management of biobanks with quality issues and benefit sharing, consent issues related to autonomy of the donors, data storage, and privacy as well as the sources and use of samples and data. Thus, one side of the coin is the many potential health benefits, such as biomarkers for clinical purposes, which makes the development of biobanks containing human samples with linkable health data ethically justifiable. The other side of the coin is the ethical costs in the form of potential loss of autonomy depending on the consent practice, unknown or even unlawful use of tissues, and their future use in ways unacceptable to people. People, in general, are interested in genetic data and willing to donate samples and data to scientific research. It is important to cherish research integrity and listen to people's opinions to retain trust. In addition to public discussion, education of both scientists and lay people, and advanced legislation are important for the ethically good long-term development for the biobanking field.

Keywords Biobanks—biorepositories—ethics—GDPR · Informed consent · Incidental findings · Dynamic consent · Biospecimen sources—autonomy—communication · Training

7.1 Introduction

Biobanks or biorepositories with human samples and related clinical data are essential starting points for modern biomedical research to pursue the etiology, molecular basis, and potential biomarkers of diseases and their treatment. Thus, the creation of

K. Vähäkangas (✉) · S. De
School of Pharmacy/Toxicology, Faculty of Health Sciences, University of Eastern Finland, Kuopio, Finland
e-mail: kirsi.vahakangas@uef.fi

P. Hainaut
Institute for Advanced Biosciences, Inserm 1209 CNRS 5309 University Grenoble-Alpes, Grenoble, France

P. Hainaut et al. (eds.), *Biobanking of Human Biospecimens*,
https://doi.org/10.1007/978-3-030-55901-4_7

biobanks is ethically justifiable. Biobanks can be disease-based, cohort biobanks (e.g., birth cohorts) as well as population biobanks and vary greatly in size, from a few hundred samples to massive ones with millions of samples [1]. A global listing of biobanks can be found at the web pages of SpecimenCentral.com which is a volunteer mediator between biobanks and scientists trying to locate proper samples for their research. In any case, the more the better applies both to the quantity of sample-data pairs giving opportunity to good statistics, as well as to the quality of samples and data for proper laboratory (high-throughput) analysis to combine with health data.

Society expects great benefits from the biobanking field, not only for the health of people but also for value creation and financial benefits [1, 2]. On the other hand, biobanks contribute to the constitution of databases of health-related personal information which, if improperly used, may cause discrimination and threaten the autonomy of persons. These benefits and risks may be mutually discrepant, forcing an ethically loaded choice within the society. For such choices to be generally understood, education is needed, and for them to be fair, general discussion based on real understanding through the education is a necessity [3]. It is, indeed, an ethical issue whether people have a real possibility to affect who decides, and how such decisions are being made. Especially, minority groups and ethnocultural communities may vary in their perception of various societal processes and would need their voice to be heard about biobanking of tissues and health data [4]. Legislation naturally is the starting point for proper conduct in society. However, although abiding by the laws is fundamental, it is often not sufficient in itself to address the broad range of issues for good research ethics, especially in the fast-developing Big Science in which biobanks play a major role [5].

Many ethical issues related to biobanks have been identified in the literature (Table 7.1; e.g., [2, 5–7]). In addition to the much discussed and obvious donor-related issues, such as informed consent, privacy, and ownership of samples, actually all aspects of biobanks have an element of ethics in the considerations whether the conduct and decisions are right or wrong, and from whose perspective. Thus, if understood widely, the ethical aspects of biobanking also include the source and use of samples, social consequences, and information of donors and communities on the development of biobanks. In this vision, all actions involved in the biobanking workflow, including the management and quality issues, have implications for ethics in addition to the protection of donors and their rights. In the literature, the most discussed ethical concerns related to biobanks and genetic research include informed consent, secondary use of genomic data and samples, de-identification and reidentification, access to the samples and data, maintenance of privacy and confidentiality, withdrawal of consent, governance, national and international collaboration, the return of results, particularly about incidental findings, as well as quality control and economic issues [1, 8–10]. Further novel ethical aspects are emerging, accelerated by the development of Artificial Intelligence and Big Data science, which makes it possible to interpolate multiple datasets to extract information that has not been explicitly identified at the onset of the project. These emerging aspects require both rigor, adaptability and creativity in applying principles of ethics to biobanking,

Table 7.1 Ethical issues of health research related to biobanks

Topic of concern	Recognized significant points	Further considerations
Source of samples	• Clinical samples • Donated samples	• Transparency of the source
Consent	• Type of consent • Understanding the consent • Autonomy • Voluntary decision-making • Ability to withdraw	• No consent • Opt-in or opt-out policy • Discontinued awareness in long-term studies
Quality issues	• Sample collection • Handling and storage conditions	• Standard operating procedure • Training of personnel
Storage and privacy	• Anonymization/coding • Retracing to donor/specific ethnic group • Access to the information • Electronic health records	• Discrimination • Stigmatization
Ownership of samples and data	• Use • Distribution	• Custodianship • Independent advisory board to decide access to and distribution of specimens • Country-specific laws on specimens
Conflicts of interest	• Economic gains of scientists	• Commercial use of donated samples
Use of samples	• Primarily research	• Consent for further use
Management of results	• Planning for disclosure • Planning for storage and future use of the result	• Incidental/secondary findings
Communication	• Education of stakeholders • Interaction between various stakeholders	• Background knowledge of different stakeholders • Different means of communication

as well as the capacity to anticipate fears and expectations as well as to react to new developments and concerns in the evolving biobanking field.

7.2 What are Biobanks?

There is no consensus on the definition of a biobank, and different authorities define a biobank in different ways and having certain common elements (Table 7.2, Fig. 7.1). Biobanks have been defined as a collection of tissue/samples and data in most of the definitions. Quite remarkably, current definitions, e.g., by MesH, ISBER, and Wikipedia refer only to storage of biological samples and do not include the associated personal and health information [15]. Although expressed in only part of the definitions, distribution of samples for various research purposes is an implicit assumption in the definitions. Where expressed the wording varies, e.g.,

Table 7.2 Definitions of biobanks—what are the essential elements?

Definitions[a]	Unique element in the definition	References
A biobank is a systematic collection of biological specimens and health information from participants		[11]
Biobanks are repositories of biological samples with accompanying linked data		[12]
A biobank is a biorepository that accepts, processes, stores, and distributes biospecimens and associated data for use in research and clinical care	Use for clinical care	[13]
Biobanks are comprehensive and well-organized collections of human biological samples and associated clinical and research data	Well-organized	[14]
Biobank is an organized collection of human biological material and associated information stored for one or more research purposes		P³G
Collections, repositories, and distribution centers of all types of human biological samples, such as blood, tissues, cells or DNA, and/or related data such as associated clinical and research data, as well as biomolecular resources, including model and microorganisms that might contribute to the understanding of the physiology and diseases of humans	Biomolecular resources, including model and microorganisms that might contribute to the understanding of the physiology and diseases of humans	BBMRI-ERIC
Facilities that collect, store, and distribute tissues—e.g., cell lines, microorganisms, blood, sperm, milk, breast tissue, for use by others. Other uses may include transplantation and comparison of diseased tissues in the identification of cancer	Uses may include transplantation	MeSH
A material entity consisting of storage facilities for specimens (DNA, blood, tissue) derived from humans and information related to these specimens		German ethics council
An entity that receives, stores, processes, and/or disseminates specimens, as needed. It encompasses the physical location as well as full range of activities associated with its operation	"Full range of activities" not defined	ISBER

P³G Public Population Project in Genomics and Society, *BBMRI-ERIC* Biobanking and BioMolecular resources Research Infrastructure-European Research Infrastructure Consortium, *MeSH* Medical subject headings, *ISBER* International Society for Biological and Environmental Repositories

[a]Direct quotations from the articles or from the organization website

"distributes" and "for use by others." Some of the definitions include also the processing of the samples ([13], ISBER (www.isber.org)). Potential commercial aspects of biobanks are not mentioned in the definitions. However, these aspects have major implications for biobanking. Beyond the potential of biobanking to support R&D and value creation, biobanking is in itself costly and financial sustainability is one of the major issues in biobanking [16–18].

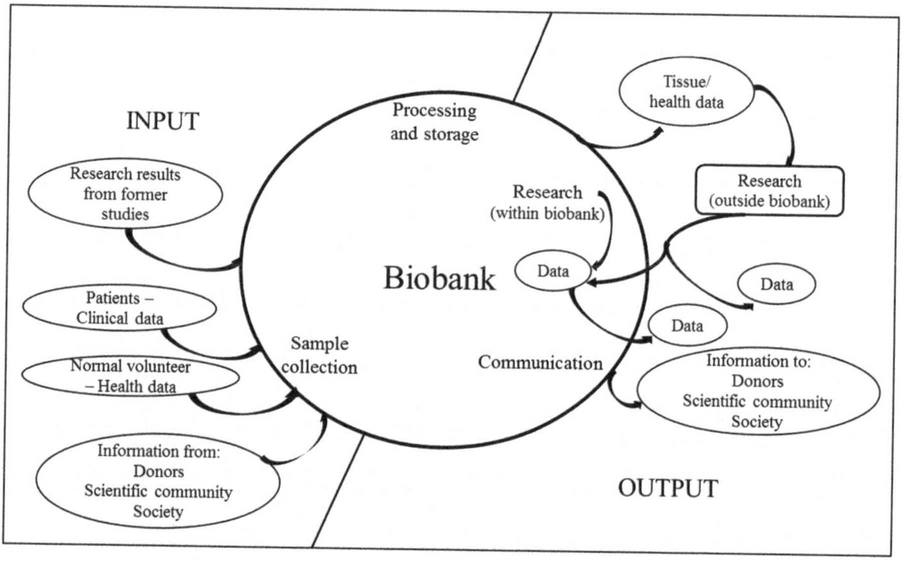

Fig. 7.1 Elements of biobank functions

Samples are physically stored in biobank facilities (repositories). This is easier for people to understand than the storage of data, which nowadays is usually made through structured electronic databases using formats that make it possible to interconnect them with each other. The weight of electronic datasets in the biobanking process is such that it is now common to conceptualize the biobanking field as a complex machinery to support the conversion of biological data into digital data through massively parallel methods such as genomics, proteomics, and metabolomics. There are different storage concepts for electronic data, none of which is fully secure, neither as to the security of data or security of privacy. Only computers not connected to the internet can be seen as relatively safe from hackers. So-called clouds, the term giving a false image of something almost out-of-reach, are just large central computers managed by some organization which probably has full access to any data in the "clouds" they manage. Protection systems, in the form of host- or network-based systems are meant to protect data from intrusion but are always, in principle, breachable. Although privacy may be overvalued, it still cannot be ethically acceptable to give people a wrong idea of the level of security of their identity linked to health data.

The various aspects of how a biobank operates are not regulated by any single legislation across Europe. However, the Council of Europe and the European Union have recommendations and regulations that are of direct relevance for biobank activities [19]. The recommendation for research on biological materials of human origin by the Council of Europe (2006) has undergone revision into the recommendation CM/Rec(2016)6 of the Committee of Ministers to member States on research on biological materials of human origin [20]. The scope of the Recommendation includes obtaining and storage of biological material of human origin for future research purposes and use of such materials for purposes other than for which they were obtained. This is however only a recommendation and not binding legislation and hence dependent on specific legislation of the Member States for its implementation.

Another relevant piece of European regulation on biobank activities is the General Data Protection Regulation (GDPR), which was applicable as of May 25, 2018 in all member states to harmonize data privacy laws across Europe. The GDPR originates from Directive 95/46 (European Parliament & European Council 1995) of European data protection law [9, 19, 21]. Being a Directive instead of a Regulation, the Member States needed to adopt it in their national law. However, a reform to the data protection rule was proposed by the European Commission in January 2012, with the release of a draft Data Protection Regulation that led to the current GDPR (Regulation (EU) 2016/- OJ L 119, 04.05.2016; cor. OJ L 127, 23.5.2018). The GDPR promotes a uniform law among the Member States. Its primary aims are to give control to individuals over their personal data and to simplify the regulatory environment for international business by unifying the regulation within the EU [22]. The GDPR also provides a regulatory framework addressing the transfer of personal data outside the EU. The GDPR is not applicable for data which are not processed and which are not identifiable. In contrast, the Recommendation CM/Rec(2016)6 considers both "identifiable" and "non-identifiable biological materials."

At the national level, only a few EU Member States have existing legislative acts specific for biobanks, such as the legislation in Iceland, Hungary, Norway, Sweden, and more recently, Finland. In other Member States, the regulatory framework for biobanks is based on the recommendations of official national bodies, formulated in reference to national laws on research on human tissues or genetic research. [23–25]. In Finland, the Biobank Act [Act 688/2012] came into force on September 1, 2013. The Act involves biobanks for all purposes, not only for biomedical research, and all samples and data in the biobanks whether identifiable or unidentifiable [24]. Until the rolling-out of the GDPR, the Directive 95/46/EC has allowed certain flexibility to the Member States in adopting it in their national law thereby leading to substantial differences among the national laws. The deployment of the GDPR now requires that Member States adapt their regulatory framework for biobanks, in particular, to take into account the specific responsibilities carried out by data controllers (including the requirement to employ a Data Protection Officer (DPO) and the so-called portability of personal data (the right for persons to obtain and carry a copy of their personal data collected by a controller in a standard format).

7.3 Management of Biobanks

In addition to the many guidelines on biobanking and its ethical aspects (Table 7.3), the literature also provides practical advice on how to establish and manage a biobank. Womack and Mager [18] list the key requirements: (1) Appropriate

Table 7.3 Organizations providing guidance and guidelines for biobanking including ethical issues

Name of the organizations	Main tasks	Websites	Relevant guidelines/ policies
Organisation for Economic Co-operation and Development (OECD)	International organization for economic development	www.oecd.org	Guidelines on Human Biobanks and Genetic Research Databases (2009)
United Nations Educational, Scientific and Cultural Organization (UNESCO)	International organization for culture and social development	www.unesco.org	1. International Declaration on Human Genetic Data (2003) 2. Universal Declaration on the Human Genome and Human Rights (1997)
Council for International Organizations of Medical Sciences (CIOMS)	International organization of biomedical scientific community also involved in developing ethical guidelines in biomedical research	www.cioms.ch	1. International Ethical Guidelines for Biomedical Research Involving Human Subjects (2002) 2. International Ethical Guidelines for Epidemiological Studies (2008)
World Medical Association (WMA)	International organization of physicians	www.wma.net	Declaration on ethical considerations regarding health databases and biobanks[a]
Council of Europe (COE)	European continent's leading human rights organization	www.coe.int	Recommendation CM/ Rec(2016)6 of the Committee of Ministers to member States on research on biological materials of human origin
Biobanking and BioMolecular resources Research Infrastructure-European Research Infrastructure Consortium (BBMRI-ERIC)	European organization for biobanks	www.bbmri-eric.eu	Common Service ELSI
Public Population Project in Genomics and Society (P^3G)	International consortium for harmonizing the functions of biobanks for population health	www.p3g.org	P^3G charter of fundamental principles

(continued)

Table 7.3 (continued)

Name of the organizations	Main tasks	Websites	Relevant guidelines/policies
International Society for Biological and Environmental Repositories (ISBER)	International organization for harmonization of biobank functions	www.isber.org	ISBER Best practices for repositories 3rd edition (Section L: legal and ethical issues for biospecimens)
Human Genome Organization (HUGO)	International organization of scientists involved in human genetics	www.hugo-international.org	Statement on Human Genomic Databases (2002)
Global Alliance for Genomics and Health (GA4GH)	International organization to create a common framework for the utilization of genomic and clinical data	www.genomicsandhealth.org	Regulatory and Ethics Working Group Work products
International Cancer Genome Consortium (ICGC)	International organization for collecting and cataloging genomic anomalies in some important cancers	www.icgc.org	Policies and guidelines on informed consent, access, and ethical oversight
US National Cancer Institute (NCI) Biorepositories and Biospecimen Research Branch (BBRB)	This is a branch of NCI (USA) providing tools for biobank functions	www.biospecimens.cancer.gov	NCI Best Practices for Biospecimen Resources

[a]A draft from the Work Group intended for open consultation after acceptance of the Executive Committee of the WMA, 18.3.2015

governance mechanisms including ethically relevant issues such as policies for consent, access and data privacy, and definitions of custodial roles and responsibilities, (2) Compliance with legal and regulatory requirements including ethical reviews and biosafety issues, also important from ethical point of view, (3) Assurance that materials are properly handled and stored, (4) Documenting the sources of human biological samples, (5) Quality control issues and accreditation, (6) Financial sustainability, and (7) Optimal usage of biobank assets, including potential use for other purposes than the ones originally planned. If a biobank company is sold or transferred to another data controller, mechanisms must be put into place to ensure that the purpose of the controller is in line with the original consent from the donors, who may have given their consent to certain type of biomedical research. Womack and Mager [18] advise that the "biobank should do everything within its powers to fulfil its contract with the subject." From an ethical point of view, sticking to the original contract with the donors would obviously be the right thing to do, but in a world driven by financial concerns this is probably just wishful thinking and binding legislation would be the only guarantee.

Organizations from different fields of interest have provided guidelines or policies which are relevant for biobank functions. Some of these organizations such as

OECD and UNESCO are large intergovernmental organizations which are not solely associated with biobanks. However, there are organizations whose primary focus is biobanks, such as ISBER and BBMRI-ERIC. Since the lack of uniform legislation regulating the functions of biobanks is well recognized, these organizations put forward guidelines for harmonizing the functioning of biobanks across Europe or internationally, thereby facilitating cross-border research which is expected to improve application of genetic and genomic research.

The more generalized guidelines such as the International Declaration on Human Genetic Data (2003) and Universal Declaration on the Human Genome and Human Rights (1997) by the UNESCO or, International Ethical Guidelines for Biomedical Research Involving Human Subjects (2002) and International Ethical Guidelines for Epidemiological Studies (2008) by CIOMS have elements which can guide the functioning of biobanks. It is however noteworthy that participant-related issues including obtaining informed consent from the participant, withdrawal of consent, and protection of privacy and confidentiality have been covered in almost all the guidelines. Apart from that, access to the samples and data, storage of samples and data, ownership of samples, benefit sharing, international collaboration, qualification and training of the personnel, standardization of procedures, disposal of samples and data have been recurring topics among the different guidelines. In UNESCO's International Declaration on Human Genetic Data (2003) and Universal Declaration on the Human Genome and Human Rights (1997), the uniqueness and sensitivity of genetic data have been highlighted. The CIOMS' guidelines on biomedical research (2002) and on epidemiological studies (2008), deal also with research in countries or communities with limited resources and issues related to externally sponsored research. There are differences in opinions on the secondary use of the collected samples among different organizations. Biobank operation requires a controlled chain of procedures, from sample and data collection to processing and storage, as well as the distribution for the most useful research. The whole operation should be sustainable operationally (requiring high-level professionals to run the biobanks), ethically (with honesty and transparency, respect for all stakeholders and their opinions, and well-informed ethics boards being involved), and economically (importance of which is supported by the development of the field of *biobankonomics*) [5, 16–18, 26]. Harmonization among biobanks would enable larger and more useful studies including rare diseases. These are very big demands achievable only through a concerted effort by various international bodies. Many international organizations, either developed for the biobanking field, such as ISBER, or existing organizations which have expanded to include biobanking in their expertise such as NCI (National Cancer Institute), part of the National Institutes of Health in the USA, provide advice on the best practices for biobanks, including ethical aspects (Table 7.3). An important resource in this respect is the International Policy interoperability and data Access Clearinghouse (IPAC) developed by the Public Population Project in Genomics and Society (P^3G), a nonprofit international consortium headed at McGill University in Montreal, Canada. The IPAC aims at proposing a "one-stop" service for harmonizing international data and biospecimen exchanges service through normative tools and frameworks that respect the laws and regulations of each country while facilitating access (http://www.p3g.org/ipac).

Issues under quality management include quality of the samples, quality management personnel, education of biobank personnel and scientists, standard operation procedures, audits or written periodic evaluations of the infrastructure, and accreditation and certification of the biobank [27]. One of the practical difficulties is retaining the quality of the samples in long-term storage. The more sensitive the molecule to be analyzed is, the more important are the storage conditions. Examples of very sensitive proteins include CYP-enzymes, which lose activity in freeze-thaw cycles [28]. Some molecules are naturally very fragile, such as RNA, while DNA can be stored long-term in many conditions. To ensure high quality and consistency of samples and their processing, a quality management system is mandatory [27]. Sample storage and processing related issues affecting the quality of the samples are, e.g., time of collection (diurnal variation), collection vessel, time from collection to processing, time from processing to freezing, temperature and length of storage, freeze-thaw cycles, and changes in SOPs over time. Naturally, all these should be carefully documented. Correct annotation of the samples requires special attention. Pellerin et al. [29] showed a 0.5% error rate among 403 DNA samples from 101 patients by analyzing four variable number of tandem repeats (VNTR). From the two mismatches found one was due to tissue mishandling and the other because of tissue mislabeling. They strongly recommend routine tissue genotyping as part of quality assurance.

Financial sustainability or biobankonomics is growing to a field in itself [1, 17]. Simeon-Dubach and Watson [1] have stressed the potential value of biobanks for all stakeholders, patients and tissue donors, funders as well as scientists. There are calculations on the start-up costs as well as the potential financial benefits, which show that the total benefits for the society would greatly outnumber the costs. The concrete products of biobanks can be in the form of publications and education, which may not bring in any immediate financial resources, but also patents and spin-off companies from the research, which can be financially evaluated. For these to materialize, more long-term investment than just for the biobank would be required. Companies are at the mercy of the world market and the possibility of people and society to pay for health. However, it is problematic if the same people try to pursue scientific truth and are responsible for the financial gain of a company. If scientists themselves stand to benefit financially from their own research there is a conflict of interest situation, which in worst case may steer the research towards less ethically sustainable practices. Examples of this have occurred in translational research for omics-based clinical biomarkers (see [5]).

7.4 The Issue of Consent

In the post-genomic era, two major changes are apparent in biomedical research: (1) the research involves minimal samples generally with less chance of physical harm to the participant and (2) the unforeseeable future use of the samples and data at the time of their collection [8, 21, 30]. The ethical concerns are aggravated by the sensitive and unique nature of the genetic information—it involves not only the donor but all those genetically related to him or her, and may reveal genotypic characteristics which are not evident phenotypically. Genetic information, if not handled properly, has the potential to discriminate and stigmatize the donor or, in certain cases, create stress and anxiety. Thus, developments in biomedical research in the post-genomic era have led to wide discussions on recognizing the ethical concerns including the consent issue in the genetic research and genomics [5, 7–10, 31]. The biobank being one of the necessary infrastructures in carrying out this research therefore comes at the forefront of ethical considerations.

Initial recognition of the requirement of informed consent in research involving human subject is included in the Guidelines for Human Experimentation of 1931, developed in pre-Nazi Germany [32, 33]. These guidelines were the first to explicitly formulate the need for "full unambiguous and informed consent from test subjects [...], except in extreme extenuating circumstances." The Nuremberg Code (1948) following the trial of the Nazi doctors and later the Declaration of Helsinki (1964, see www.wma.net) further established the concept of protecting the research subject by prioritizing his or her well-being over the advancement of science and society and by clearly stressing the need for a formal informed consent. The Declaration of Helsinki represents a foundation for biomedical research and constitutes a cornerstone for many legal frameworks across the world [8, 34]. The concept of informed consent has two important aspects—autonomy and information. The purpose of informed consent is to provide the research subjects with adequate information about the research, including possible harms and benefits, before obtaining a voluntary, autonomous decision of participation from them. All in all, the ethical considerations in various existing guidelines and legislations are based on the idea of traditional research where the primary concern was physical harm to the research participant.

In biobanking, the unique challenge as compared to traditional research projects is that the exact destination and usage of the collected samples and data are not always known at the time of collection. Hence, the type of consent that is most suitable for biobanks has been a topic of wide discussion and is still debated in the literature. The types of consents mentioned in the literature for biomedical research are specific consent, and broader consent types such as sectoral consent, blanket consent, or open consent [21, 30, 35]. These have implications as to the amount of autonomy of the research participant (Fig. 7.2). In the current practice of biobanks, however, the most common type of consent in use is broad consent [35]. The main difference between specific consent and broad consent is the information, or lack of it, provided to the donor at the time of collection about the possible uses of the samples and data. Since informed consent is supposed to include detailed information of various aspects of the research including how the samples or data will be used, it can be argued that a broad consent which does not provide such information is not an informed consent at all [36]. Similarly, the use of a presumed consent with the provision to opt-out has also been debated intensely on the same grounds [37–40].

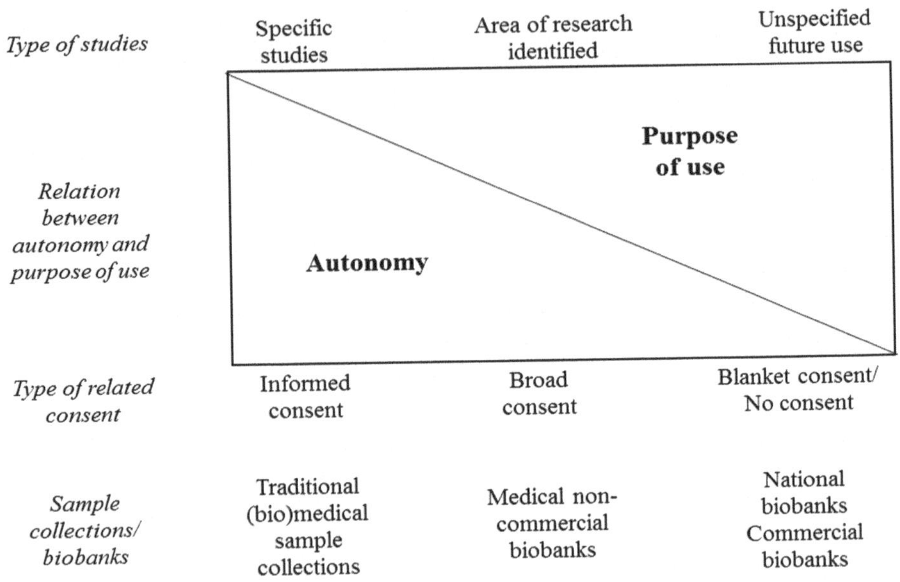

Fig. 7.2 Degree of autonomy in relation to other aspects of biobanking

Another consent type which is gaining support in the context of biobanks is the dynamic consent. Dynamic consent involves providing and updating information to the donors and putting them in control for the use of their samples or data, through a web-based platform, and has been argued to be more suited for biobanks compared to other consent types [41]. The term "dynamic consent" was coined by Jane Kaye of the University of Oxford in the course of the EnCoRe project (Ensuring Consent and Revocation), a joint academy-industry program developed in the UK between 2008 and 2012 to explore new mechanisms for empowering individuals with more control over any personal data they disclose, with the overall vision of making the consent "as reliable and easy as turning on a tap, and revoking that consent as reliable and easy as turning it off again." EnCoRe included research on the development of appropriate regulatory regimes, on IT system architectures, on consent management systems, and on the development and implementation of easy-to-use interfaces and has released publicly available deliverables on each of these aspects (https://www.hpl.hp.com/breweb/encoreproject/deliverables.html). An interesting idea emerged from the studies by Conley et al. [42], who concluded that the opinions of the research participants in biobank studies about their samples and the conditions of their use resembled a trade secret concept. Based on this, they propose a legal contract as the basis of the exchange of their DNA to compensation and/or information. This actually resembles the situation of the company 23andME which provides genetic information in exchange for a saliva sample (Box 7.1). When people feel that they are in the control and can decide for themselves, they seem to be very open to providing samples and data for research.

Criticisms of dynamic consent have argued that such an extensive form of participation is not necessary. A systematic analysis of the qualitative sociological literature on public and patient's perceptions towards consent concluded that "few people demanded recurrent, project-specific consent." Other criticisms have argued that dynamic consent may actually cause bias for recruiting study participants by repeatedly confronting them to the complexity of biomedical research and asking them again and again to formulate an "opinion." However, as public perceptions evolve over time, and as individuals become more and more aware of their rights and of the need to protect their personal data, the concept of dynamic consent is gaining traction, in particular, for prospective studies.

In the Data Protection Regulation [22], processing of special data including genetic and health data is only possible in certain cases as listed in Article 9 (2). The first point mentioned in this list (Article 9 (2) (a)) is to obtain a consent from the donor, followed by other situations (Article 9 (2) (b–j)) where processing of genetic data is possible even without the donor's consent. In this regard, Hallinan and Friedewald [21] have presented justifications for the absolute necessity of a consent from donors for biobanks, to uphold the ethical principle of autonomy in biomedical research and to maintain the fundamental rights of the person providing the data. The information to be provided to the sample donor when the data and samples are directly collected from the donor are listed in Article 13 of the Data Protection Regulation. Apart from other information, the purpose of processing, the period of storage, restrictions to processing, and the right to withdraw consent at any time are mentioned in the list. An important aspect in the consent issue is the fact that people have difficulties in understanding and remembering what they have consented to [43] stressing the quality of information given to participants as well as enough time to consider and discuss with other people [36].

With the development of Artificial Intelligence and the exponential growth of opportunities to aggregate health-related personal data with multiple other data sources, new mechanisms should be considered to ensure the rights of individuals to retain control over their personal data. Among such mechanisms, citizen-owned nonprofit data cooperatives may provide a basis for a democratically controlled and fair personal data ecosystem from which society at large may benefit. Cooperatives imply participatory forms of governance that set them aside from other forms of organizations such as foundations or shareholder-owned companies. A prototype for such a model is the Midata platform, a citizen-owned nonprofit cooperative founded in Switzerland in 2015 with the aim of acting as a trustee for data collection and guaranteeing the sovereignty of citizens over the use of their data. Within this model, individuals actively contribute to research as users of the platform by providing access to data sets and as cooperative members to control and develop the cooperative (https://www.midata.coop/en/home/).

7.5 Sources and Use of Tissues and Data

The multiple possible sources of tissue samples have different implications for the donor. Samples can be directly collected specifically to the biobank. However, the collection of samples can also be left-over tissue from surgery, or laboratory samples collected for medical tests, or from tissue biopsies, or from pathology archives. An interesting case is the company 23andME which retains samples and data from commercial genetic testing of customers (Box 7.1). Samples collected for biobanks are of different nature, from simple saliva samples from normal volunteers apparently with no health risk to the donor, as in the case of the kit sold by the 23andME company [44] to serial biopsies from tumor tissue with potential harm to the patient [45]. The risks of such biopsies include hemorrhage, infection, and needle-track

Box 7.1 The Case of 23andMe

The company 23andMe started off in 2006 as a genetic testing company providing direct-to-consumer testing [44]. In addition to selling tests to consumers, it developed a parallel business of selling tissues and data to scientific research. Consumers of the tests were asked to provide health information, access to their Internet behavior and requested to fill in an informed consent to use their left-over samples for research. The trust of genetic testing as a business opportunity was proven by the investments raised: by September 2012 the company had collected over 100 million US $, Google being the biggest investor. By 2016 their biobank contained DNA samples, related health data, and consent for further research from over four million people.

In practice, the company sells online kits to collect a saliva sample. The sample is shipped to the company and tested for two million whole genome SNPs, including SNPs associated with susceptibility to diseases. The customer receives a report through a personal web account. The rest of the sample is stored to be sold for public or private-supported research if the customer has signed a consent. Customers are attracted to this possibility by presenting it as a "full service" providing extra information. Of note, the extent of collected information goes far beyond self-reported health information, also including web behavior, no doubt interesting to advertising companies.

Future plans include consumer health service and a drug discovery program [80]. After a warning by FDA in 2013 about non-validated health-related genetic tests, the company is now collaborating with the FDA in developing health reports and getting them to the customers. In the meantime, the FDA has approved a genetic test for susceptibility to Bloom's syndrome. Drug discovery is a logical expansion of the business, from SNPs to sequencing and from known associations to new druggable target identification. In the words of the platform architect Arnab Chowdry: "having it in-house means that we get a bigger chunk of the value" (quote from [80]). According to Servick, people provide their data to 23andME willingly, being "almost addicted to participating in research."

seeding of the tumor, which are said to be extremely rare. Basik et al. [45], however, mention that safety data from cancer biopsies is scarce and the risks not fully understood. Despite these limitations, ethics review boards have generally considered favorably research projects involving serial tumor biopsies in clinical trials because the benefit to society outweighs the risk to an individual patient [45, 46]. Such thinking is not in line with the Declaration of Helsinki which states that society and scientific research should never be put above the safety of a patient. The source of samples naturally has a lot of implications for the contents of the informed consent, which needs to list potential risks to the donor. It is important to realize that sick patients may misunderstand sampling for research with sampling for clinical purposes (the so-called therapeutic misconception which is highly debated, e.g. [47]).

Human tissue are invaluable resources both in research and in clinical medicine. It is no wonder then that tissue procurement for research has sometimes taken unethical turns, especially when stakes are high, health-wise and/or financially. The example of illegal organ trafficking in transplant business (Box 7.2) makes it clear

Box 7.2 Unethical Organ Trade

Improving organ transplantation practices since 1990 have led to increasing demands of transplantable organs. The business opportunity was immediately recognized by international criminal networks and illegal organ trade started to bloom. This was made possible by corrupt medical doctors and surgeons, public and private insurance companies paying costs of transplant operations abroad without checking the source of organs, and poverty among people willing to risk their health and life against donations, most of the time ignorant of the implications (see, e.g., [49, 90, 91]). In China, involuntary organ harvesting is forbidden by law but a 1984 regulation made it legal to remove organs from executed criminals with their prior consent or consent from relatives. It has been alleged that in 2006, 4000 executed prisoners provided thousands of kidneys and livers for mainly foreign patients [48]. The practice has been recognized by Chinese authorities and in 2007, China issued new regulation banning organ trade. Despite this, consistent media reports suggest that the practice still continues. In India, legal loopholes and poverty turned the country into a large market of kidney transplants. Poor people were often lured and forced by false promises to donate organs. Stricter regulations were put into place in 1994 but there is evidence that organized networks still evade these legal restrictions to continue organ trade. A survey in India showed that a significantly higher percentage of the sellers were under poverty line after the surgery than before, and up to a half were having health issues from the surgery [92]. Iran is the only country where organ trade is legal [92]. The trade is controlled by charity organizations with government support. Despite provided health insurance and heavy regulation to protect the donors, most of them, when asked afterwards would not do it again or recommend selling an organ.

(continued)

Box 7.2 (continued)

"Transplant tourism" (TT) consists of sick people from rich countries traveling to less developed countries in order to seek commercial transplantation opportunities. Efrat [93] compared the situation in two countries, Israel and Pakistan, both of which changed their legislation after the Declaration of Istanbul on Organ Trafficking and Transplant Tourism in 2008 [94]. In a few years in Israel, TT decreased significantly to one-fifth, while in Pakistan the changed legislation did not have a clear effect. Difficulties in cutting TT related to a large number of middlemen financially benefitting from organ trade. The fact that some countries do not release precise statistics makes monitoring the global situation impossible. From global ethical point of view, it is difficult to accept different local ethical standards for commercial organ transplantation [95] or regulated reimbursement model to increase living donations [90], as has been suggested as a solution to the lack of transplantable organs.

that criminal sources of tissue are difficult to eliminate and sometimes almost impossible to trace. Despite the internationally agreed Istanbul Declaration to stop organ trafficking [48], the practice remains underreported and has not stopped [49]. Concerns regarding "tissues for sale" are an important ethical issue, in particular, when biobanks are run as commercial, for-profit organizations. These concerns underscore the need for both public discussion of all aspects of biobanks and transparency about the sources of tissue.

Biobanks may be designed to serve different purposes, some of which are generally regarded as ethically good, such as the conservation of natural variations of species or the promotion of human health. However, within the medical field, opinions may vary regarding the acceptability of specific biobanking practices. For instance, there are different views on how to deal with genetic testing on fetuses and its implications. Testing for life-threatening genetic aberrations is probably acceptable to most people and justifies biobanking. The availability of both genetic tests and biobank infrastructure raises an ethical challenge in providing opportunities for extending testing to conditions that do not dramatically reduce the quality of life of the person (e.g., Down syndrome; [50]). In the study by Hill et al. [51] the parents pointed out two important points in prenatal genetic testing for single gene diseases: the accuracy of the test and the availability of genetic counseling in connection with the testing.

A particular ethical challenge arises when a biobank has to cease its activity and to face closure and dispersion of its contents. It is striking to note that many regulations and guidelines have been developed on how to build a biobank and that almost none address the difficult problem of biobank closure. Whether or not specimens and data should be simply disposed of and destroyed at the end of a specific program is a matter of debate, with arguments for both sides of the coin. When decisions of retaining specimens are made, they must be transferred to another biobank and repurposed for other programs. There are no defined ethical guidelines regulating such decision processes. The problem is compounded when biobanks face unscheduled closure due to lack of funding, technical problems, or lack of appropriate governance. In such cases, a conservative approach would require that a biobank closure program be formally developed and submitted for approval by a relevant legal or institutional ethical review board. Biobanks should consider insuring themselves against the risk of unexpected closure in order to make sure they have sufficient resources to handle the ethical dispersion of their assets.

Finally, one should keep in mind that it is always possible to use tissues and data from biobanks for sinister purposes, as well. Recent history is rife with discrimination based on skin color, ethnicity, or, indeed, diseases. For instance, mentally incapacitated or ill, and patients with epilepsy were force-sterilized according to law until to the late 1960 in the USA and Europe, including Finland, a practice now regarded as totally unacceptable and criminal (see, e.g., [52, 53]). It is not far-fetched to imagine that someone somewhere given the chance, e.g., by non-existing oversight of further use of the samples and data, would buy the material for purposes not generally acceptable. Examples include development of targeted biological weapons or discrimination based on ethnicity in the war zones.

7.6 Incidental Findings

In high-throughput genetic analysis such as genome wide sequencing (GWS) or whole exome/genome sequencing (WES) the amount of achieved information is staggering. Such studies are usually designed as exploratory endeavors attempting to find links between phenotypes or disease and genomic traits. In the course of such analyses, gene variants are found which are known or suspected to associate with conditions and diseases other than those under study [54, 55]. Such incidental or secondary findings (IF) create ethical issues that need to be considered in any biobank-based study [56–60]. It is recognized that biobanks should include in their policy a strategy for the documentation, management, and communication of incidental findings. Naturally, individual differences occur in opinions, even among professionals whether to whom and how to give information of genomic variations and their relationship with diseases or disease risk [61]. Arguments both for and against giving out the individual findings can be presented (Table 7.4). For these reasons, Viberg et al. [57] call for more empirical research before comprehensive policy for handling incidental findings in biobank research is adopted.

A list of existing guidelines and laws outside the US on return of individual research results (IRRs) and IFs are given by Zawati and Knoppers [62]. Among the 15 documents, three are legal documents, the rest being guidelines and hence not legally binding. In spite of this, a lack of sufficient guidance in the literature for managing and returning IFs in genomic biobank research is noted by Wolf et al. [58] and Wolf [63]. Wolf et al. [58] report recommendations developed in an NIH-funded

Table 7.4 Arguments for and against delivery of incidental findings in biobank studies (based partly on [57]

	Considerations	Whose interest
Arguments for		
Disclosure is beneficial for individuals	Is the result analytically valid, clinically significant, and actionable	Participant, family, society
Disclosure promotes autonomy	Do the results have clear clinical use. Are they important to life decisions	Participant
Reciprocity requires disclosure	Participant gives a sample and gets information of his/her genetic status in return	Participant, scientist, research group
Return of incidental findings is in accordance with participant's wishes	Many or even most people want to receive individual genetic information	Participant
Arguments against		
Practical issues make disclosure unfeasible	Difficult to find a solution that fits all, risk of breaching confidentiality if all information of participants retained	Scientist, research group, participant
Disclosure can harm participants	Therapeutic misconception, potential anxiety, accidental delivery of wrong information	Participant, family, health care professionals
The relationship between scientist and participant does not create duty	Difference between a scientist and a clinical doctor	Scientist
Disclosure can harm research and prevent research from doing good	Beneficence in research is at collective level while in care at individual level	Research group, scientist, society

project, where they have identified biobank as the hub of a "biobank research system" that includes the primary research sites (collection sites) and the secondary research sites where biobank samples and associated data are processed and analyzed. The ten recommendations put forward by these authors highlight the central responsibility of the biobank itself in the management and return of IFs and IRRs. The differences in challenges between the preexisting and new biobanks in executing these recommendations have also been discussed, as well as the costs involved in returning IRRs and IFs [64].

A major question about IFs and IRRs is to determine which results and information should be returned to study participants [61, 65–68]. Wolf and coworkers [58] have categorized IFs into those which should be returned, could be returned, and should not be returned to the contributors (providers of samples and data). The IFs that should be returned are the analytically valid IFs of a serious health condition with substantial risk which are actionable and satisfy the applicable law (for example, verification from a CLIA certified laboratory). The IFs which could be returned are those which satisfy all the abovementioned criteria except being actionable but yet having "established and substantial risk of likely health or reproductive importance or personal utility […] likely to provide net benefit from the contributor's perspective." The IFs without personal utility or clinical significance are suggested not to be returned.

Very few original studies have addressed the perceptions of people about delivering individual genetic information to the donors of samples. Indeed, the wide variety of situations make it impossible to define a uniform approach. Aspects to consider include the situation of the individual (patient or non-patient volunteer), age and status (adult, fetus or child, non-autonomous persons), and clinical significance of the incidental finding (disease marker vs. risk for disease; childhood-onset vs. adult-onset disease; whether it is treatable or not). For a lay person, the notion of risk is often unclear and people may easily confuse an incidental disease with incidentally found risk for disease [57]. "Therapeutic misconception" is a term used by Appelbaum et al. [69] to describe the situation when people "fail[ed] to appreciate the distinction between the imperatives of clinical research and of ordinary treatment." Therapeutic misconception has been mentioned in the context of participant's expectations regarding the return of genomic IRRs and IFs [62, 70]. Townsend et al. [71] have reported that the general public and the parents of children with intellectual disabilities, who have undergone genetic testing with inconclusive results, were of the opinion that they should have a say in deciding what results should be disclosed to them. They regarded personal choice as more important than clinical relevance. A similar attitude was also observed in a study by Clift et al. [72], where patients and family members undergoing clinical genomic sequencing felt that they should be able to take part in the decision-making process about which results should be returned to them. In another study, a majority of lung and colorectal cancer patients stated their desire to be informed of all types of results, including genetic IFs [73]. On the other hand, genetic professionals often prefer to restrain the volume of data to be processed and to be selective on what and when to give to patients [74]. In the opinion of most genetic professionals, excessive data can be useless and stressful to the patient, in addition to requiring a lot of wasted resources. The authors point to knowledge in genetics as one of the potential reasons for such difference between the opinions of laypersons and professionals [75, 76].

From a biobanking perspective, the ethical challenges raised by IFs are important because the true significance of an IF may become apparent only several years after the completion of a research project. In this context, the biobank fulfills its role as a hub of a "biobank research system" by acting as a repository for information that patients and participants may feel of relevance to them. Although autonomy is encouraged legally and ethically, any decision of giving such information should be made after thorough consideration and understanding of the available information and not just mechanically exercising one's right.

7.7 Communication and Education

In recent years the development of high-throughput "omics" methodologies such as genomics, proteomics, or metabolomics, coupled with enhanced computing power and artificial intelligence, have propelled biomedical into a new era of "big data science." This new form of large-scale biology provides an unprecedented volume of information on individual variations associated with health status, but also raises a number of ethical challenges (e.g., [5]). The aggregation of high-throughput data, made possible by linkable sample sets provided by biobanks, is essential for the development of clinical biomarkers and for drug development. Thus, it is no wonder that there is a lot of hype and enthusiasm on the role of biobanks in clinical research, both from the ethical perspective of advancing treatment and care, and from the ethically more complex perspective of making financial profit. This complex set-up makes communication and dialog mandatory between various stakeholders: (1) among scientists, (2) between scientists and participants providing tissues and data, (3) between scientists and investors either public or private, providing funding for research, and (4) between scientists, the public, decision-makers, and the society as a whole, who should ultimately exert the final say on these decisions. Successful communication between different stakeholders in biobanking requires education to understand the concepts and implications of large-scale biology, as well as the specific requirements of biobanking in this respect. Both nonprofessionals as tissue donors and participants in scientific projects to understand what they consent to, as well as people taking part in decision-making, e.g., when designing new legislation, need a sound understanding of biobanking issues and ethical challenges.

From the scientist's perspective, education and training are fundamental to correctly identify and duly address the various ethical challenges of biobanking and large-scale research in developing a research project. This has very practical implications, e.g., when submitting a protocol to an ethics committee or when preparing a grant application. Good communication between scientists is especially challenging in international multidisciplinary fields such as biobanking. Thus, it is important to know about the history and cultural differences to avoid past mistakes [3, 5]. Scientists themselves start to realize the importance and need of education in ethics [5, 36, 77] and the best ways of ethics teaching are actively investigated [78]. When stakes are high and scientific competition intense, multiple dangers arise, such as hastily-drawn or reductive translational studies on immature biomarkers, conflicts of interest between stakeholders (patients, researchers, industry), and temptation to cut corners in science, causing misconduct (e.g., [79]). Research integrity should be promoted by all means in the midst of enthusiasm. Although formal education in ethics of young scientists is required, the example by senior scientists through model learning is probably the most effective way [5]. No ethics teaching will sustain good scientific practice if research institutions, academia, and scientific journals do not create an appropriate context for research integrity and provide means to deal with scientific misconduct (as an example of recommendations on how to deal with research misconduct see www.tenk.fi).

Communication with the public is being made simple by easy access to the Internet. Both invitations to participate in research and biobanks and information distribution can be efficiently carried out through the internet. Although this possibility is already utilized in scientific research, there are limits: older people may not be computer literate or have a computer, and literacy or connection to the Internet is not self-evident in all parts of the world. An ethically relevant issue is also the behavior of people, which changes according to the situation and is more relaxed at the computer than face-to-face. In fact, for some commercial companies, it has appeared very easy to get health data directly from people through Internet questionnaires [80].

Due to decreasing costs of genome sequencing, direct-to-consumer genetic testing (DTC-GT) is turning into a thriving business (for reviews see, e.g., [81, 82]). A flagship in this business is 23andMe, a US-based company ([44]; see Box 7.1) which has created a two-way business by selling genetic testing over the Internet and then asking for consent to retain the rest of the samples which are then sold further. Their biobank with matched samples and data is one of the largest existing. Thus, in this business model, the consumer (a healthy volunteer from the point of view of research) does not communicate with a doctor, nor with a scientist, but with a multinational commercial company. As pointed out by Zawati et al. [83], this is not unique to this company, and other DTC-GT companies often retain data from the analysis for future use.

When dealing with DTC-GT companies the privacy and autonomy of the consumers end when they fill out the health data sheet and sign the consent. They do not have any control over the purpose their samples are sold for. In the literature, the concerns on the adequacy of the consumer's consent and the transparency of the direct-to-consumer genetic testing companies have been expressed based on the data given in the company web pages, the only places where consumers can find information, often insufficient and even misleading [84], before making the decision whether to subject their DNA for testing [85]. Furthermore, many of the companies, based on their web pages, may not have clear policies as to testing of children, an issue where professional scientific researchers and organizations have made a significant effort creating guidelines [86].

The uniqueness of genetic data is well recognized in the literature and legislation. Unfortunately, the general public may not be aware of it and often lack the necessary knowledge to understand the future implications of sending their samples and personal information for such tests, and the information provided in many cases is not of sufficient help [84]. The absence of a health care professional to provide an overview of the process has led to this gap of knowledge and understanding which is being utilized by the DTC-GT companies for their commercial gains. The many ethical issues recognized in the literature regarding DTC-GT include misleading commercials, lack of reliability of tests, future use of the samples and data, what happens to the samples and data when these companies shut down, emotional impact to the customers on receiving the results, and tests for newborn or children. The bigger the company, the more share of the market it is able to buy and such a monopoly can be regarded even as a possible threat to democracy [44].

7.8 Conclusion

In biomedical research, good ethics is based on three basic ideas: honesty, respect, and professionalism. The generally accepted starting point is the value of human life. Even if these were self-evident in various functions of society, including medical research, healthcare, and biobanking, a lot of developmental work and negotiations between stakeholders are needed in proper implementation of these principles. Multiple factors, such as the pursuit of personal or private interests, misuse of opportunities for financial gain and fame, carelessness in practical work, ignorance of proper rules of practice, or inappropriate use of biobanked tissues and data may compromise good ethical practice. Moreover, even when the intentions are good, quality pursued, and professional demands respected, there is always a possibility of human error. It is ethically important to admit this and make plans to deal with such flaws.

The basic dilemma of medical ethics lies in the difficulty to take into account both sides of the same coin. One side of the coin is the great expected health benefits from studies using human tissues. The other side is the ethical costs, in the form of potential harm for participants, loss of autonomy, unknown or even criminal use or sale of human tissue, and commercial use of tissues in a way unacceptable by people. The activities of biobanks actually place them precisely at the tipping point where the coin may flip towards one side or the other. In terms of ethical impact, biobanks have two characteristics that make them particularly important. First, they are durable (they generally exceed the lifetime of the projects they support and even the career of the scientist who has created them). This implies that biobanks are the most evident point of entry for secondary or tertiary usage of stored tissues, which can take place years if not decades after the initial tissue and data collection. Second, they operate at a critical junction in science, where biological data are processed and transformed into digital data. This particular role places biobanks with the specific responsibility of acting as custodian and caretaker for huge volumes of "data-to-be," the significance and impact of which is very difficult to predict. Despite these characteristics, biobanks are often merely considered just as technical infrastructure in the design and ethical approval of studies using human tissues. They are evaluated on the basis of their technical performance and compliance with recommended standards for specimen processing and storage. Their ethical responsibilities in setting up appropriate mechanisms and safeguards for long-term access and usage of tissues are rarely challenged. With the growing interoperability of multiple data sources, the ethical responsibilities of biobanks, both as data sources and custodians, will come under further scrutiny and will need to be addressed by appropriate regulation and legislation.

Ethics is about making balanced choices in particular in "grey zones" where regulation and legislation are underdeveloped or inexistent. As highlighted throughout this chapter, ethics for biobanks still contain many such "grey zones" and is therefore an important field for research and debate. Incidental/secondary findings, not explicitly targeted by initial research protocols but appearing as additional findings in large-scale molecular analyses, are unavoidable [87, 88]. Variants with no significance at the time of analysis may appear significant by time, which makes the accuracy of the analysis and proper documentation of the findings important. Strategy on whether and how to inform participants about secondary findings and what kind of support to give to those who find out or are told about a significant secondary finding should be in place beforehand.

Advancing this field of ethics for biobanks should be built on several pillars: (1) transparency enabled by education and public discussion, aimed at making participants, actors, and stakeholders knowledgeable about biobanking processes and ethical implications; (2) good governance, aiming at making participants an integral part of decision processes regarding tissue and data usage; (3) sound and fair funding and business models, ensuring the long-term viability of high-quality biobanks and protecting them against many forms of misuse that may stem from insufficient resources.

Human nature is somewhat irrational and unfortunately also susceptible to corruption. Institutions and organizations are not eternal and when they fail or die, their assets are often left to grabs according to market laws. When money becomes the main or the only driving force, many good principles may be forgotten or overruled. From a purely business point of view, quick, easy, and cheap access to data and tissue are the primary interest. From this point of view, regulations are often perceived as obstacles for innovation and value creation. However, from the point of view of respect for the participants and addressing the expectations of society as a whole, things look different. Fair regulation protects people and also provides a framework for good science oriented towards benefits for the people. Good societal ethics requires the protection of those less privileged and democratic decision systems to ensure the use of tissues and data in biobanks for generally acceptable purposes. Biobanks can be seen as giant telescopes for biomedical research, operating as large instruments that can be pointed towards unexplored areas of the deep universe of human biology. By transmuting the codes of Nature into digital data, biobanks operate at the very interface between Nature and Culture. We need a model where best practice from a technical viewpoint can make a harmonious match with the best practice from an ethical viewpoint [89]. This would not take away passion, intensity, and contradiction from the ethical scientific debate, but would outline a pragmatic road ahead for addressing the scientific and societal challenges and opportunities of "big data" research using human tissues.

Accepting the existence of issues and bringing them into awareness are the initial steps in establishing good ethical practices. In this chapter, we have pointed out the "grey zones" in biobanking and described the background for their existence. Such discussion, we hope, moves the biobanking field closer to building the best ethical practices.

References

1. Simeon-Dubach D, Watson P (2014) Biobanking 3.0: evidence based and customer focused biobanking. Clin Biochem 47:300–308
2. Carter A, Betsou F (2011) Quality assurance in cancer biobanking. Biopreserv Biobank 9:157–163
3. Wright GE, Koornhof PG, Adeyemo AA, Tiffin N (2013) Ethical and legal implications of whole genome and whole exome sequencing in African populations. BMC Med Ethics 14:21

4. Godard B, Ozdemir V, Fortin M, Egalité N (2010) Ethnocultural community leaders' views and perceptions on biobanks and population specific genomic research: a qualitative research study. Public Underst Sci. 19:469–485
5. Vähäkangas K (2013) Research ethics in the post-genomic era. Environ Mol Mutagen 54:599–610
6. Kinkorová J (2015) Biobanks in the era of personalized medicine: objectives, challenges, and innovation. EPMA J 7:4
7. Scott CT, Caulfield T, Borgelt E, Illes J (2012) Personal medicine—the new banking crisis. Nat Biotechnol 30:141–147
8. Melham K, Moraia LB, Mitchell C, Morrison M, Teare H, Kaye J (2014) The evolution of withdrawal: negotiating research relationships in biobanking. Life Sci Soc Policy 10:16
9. Thorogood A, Zawati MH (2015) International guidelines for privacy in genomic biobanking (or the unexpected virtue of pluralism). J Law Med Ethics 43:690–702
10. Virani AH, Longstaff H (2015) Ethical considerations in biobanks: how a public health ethics perspective sheds new light on old controversies. J Genet Couns 24:428–432
11. Olson JE, Bielinski SJ, Ryu E, Winkler EM, Takahashi PY, Pathak J, Cerhan JR (2014) Biobanks and personalized medicine. Clin Genet. 86:50–55
12. Shaw DM, Elger BS, Colledge F (2014) What is a biobank? Differing definitions among biobank stakeholders. Clin Genet. 85:223–227
13. De Souza YG, Greenspan JS (2013) Biobanking past, present and future: responsibilities and benefits. AIDS 27(3):303–312
14. Harris JR, Burton P, Knoppers BM, Lindpaintner K, Bledsoe M, Brookes AJ, Budin-Ljøsne I, Chisholm R, Cox D, Deschênes M, Fortier I, Hainaut P, Hewitt R, Kaye J, Litton JE, Metspalu A, Ollier B, Palmer LJ, Palotie A, Pasterk M, Perola M, Riegman PH, van Ommen GJ, Yuille M, Zatloukal K (2012) Toward a roadmap in global biobanking for health. Eur J Hum Genet. 20:1105–1101
15. Fransson MN, Rial-Sebbag E, Brochhausen M, Litton JE (2015) Toward a common language for biobanking. Eur J Hum Genet 23:22–28
16. De Souza YG (2015) Sustainability of biobanks in the future. Adv Exp Med Biol 864:29–35
17. Vaught J, Rogers J, Carolin T, Compton C (2011) Biobankonomics: developing a sustainable business model approach for the formation of a human tissue biobank. J Natl Cancer Inst Monogr 2011:24–31
18. Womack C, Mager SR (2014) Human biological sample biobanking to support tissue biomarkers in pharmaceutical research and development. Methods 70:3–11
19. Townend D (2016) EU Laws on privacy in genomic databases and biobanking. J Law Med Ethics 44:128–142
20. Council of Europe (2016) Recommendation CM/Rec(2016)6 of the Committee of Ministers to member States on research on biological materials of human origin. https://search.coe.int/cm/Pages/result_details.aspx?ObjectId=090000168064e8ff. Accessed 10 Jul 2016
21. Hallinan D, Friedewald M (2015) Open consent, biobanking and data protection law: can open consent be 'informed' under the forthcoming data protection regulation? Life Sci Soc Policy 11:1
22. European Commission (2016) Reform of EU data protection rules. http://ec.europa.eu/justice/data-protection/reform/index_en.htm. Accessed 10 Jul 2016
23. European Commission (2012) Biobanks for Europe A challenge for governance. https://ec.europa.eu/research/swafs/pdf/pub_archive/biobanks-for-europe_en.pdf. Accessed 10 Jul 2016
24. Soini S (2013) Finland on a road towards a modern legal biobanking infrastructure. Eur J Health Law 20:289–294
25. Zawati MH, Knoppers B, Thorogood A (2014) Population biobanking and international collaboration. Pathobiology 81:276–285
26. Parry-Jones A (2014) Assessing the financial, operational, and social sustainability of a biobank: the Wales Cancer Bank case study. Biopreserv Biobank 12:381–388

27. Grizzle WE, Gunter EW, Sexton KC, Bell WC (2015) Quality management of biorepositories. Biopreserv Biobank 13:183–194
28. Yamazaki H, Inoue K, Turvy CG, Guengerich FP, Shimada T (1997) Effects of freezing, thawing, and storage of human liver samples on the microsomal contents and activities of cytochrome P450 enzymes. Drug Metab Dispos 25:168–174
29. Pellerin C, McKercher G, Aprikian AG, Saad F, Lacombe L, Carmel M, Chevalier S (2016) A simple variable number of tandem repeat-based genotyping strategy for the detection of handling errors and validation of sample identity in biobanks. Biopreserv Biobank 14(5):383–389. [Epub ahead of print]
30. Helgesson G (2012) In defense of broad consent. Camb Q Healthc Ethics 21:40–50
31. Egalite N, Groisman IJ, Godard B (2014) Genetic counseling practice in next generation sequencing research: implications for the ethical oversight of the informed consent process. J Genet Couns 23:661–670
32. Ghooi RB (2011) The Nuremberg Code-A critique. Perspect Clin Res 2:72–76
33. Sade RM (2003) Publication of unethical research studies: the importance of informed consent. Ann Thorac Surg 75:325–328
34. Vähäkangas K (2001) Ethical implications of genetic analysis of individual susceptibility to diseases. Mutat Res 482:105–110
35. Master Z, Nelson E, Murdoch B, Caulfield T (2012) Biobanks, consent and claims of consensus. Nat Methods 9:885–888
36. Vähäkangas K (2004) Ethical aspects of molecular epidemiology of cancer. Carcinogenesis 25:465–471
37. Arnason V (2004) Coding and consent: moral challenges of the database project in Iceland. Bioethics 18:27–49
38. Caulfield T, Upshur RE, Daar A (2003) DNA databanks and consent: a suggested policy option involving an authorization model. BMC Med Ethics 4:E1
39. Caulfield T (2007) Biobanks and blanket consent: the proper place of the public good and public perception rationales. Kings Law J 18:209–226
40. Hofmann B (2009) Broadening consent—and diluting ethics? J Med Ethics 35:125–129
41. Kaye J, Whitley EA, Lund D, Morrison M, Teare H, Melham K (2015) Dynamic consent: a patient interface for twenty-first century research networks. Eur J Hum Genet 23(2):141–146
42. Conley JM, Kenan WR, Mitchell R, Cadigan RJ, Davis AM, Dobson AW, Gladden RQ (2012) A trade secret model for genomic biobanking. J Law Med Ethics 40:612–629
43. D'Abramo F, Schildmann J, Vollmann J (2015) Research participants' perceptions and views on consent for biobank research: a review of empirical data and ethical analysis. BMC Med Ethics 16:60
44. Stoeklé HC, Mamzer-Bruneel MF, Vogt G, Hervé C (2016) 23andMe: a new two-sided data-banking market model. BMC Med Ethics 17:19
45. Basik M, Aguilar-Mahecha A, Rousseau C, Diaz Z, Tejpar S, Spatz A, Greenwood CM, Batist G (2013) Biopsies: next-generation biospecimens for tailoring therapy. Nat Rev Clin Oncol 10:437–450
46. Lee JM, Hays JL, Noonan AM, Squires J, Minasian L, Annunziata C, Wood BJ, Yu M, Calvo KR, Houston N, Azad N, Kohn EC (2013) Feasibility and safety of sequential research-related tumor core biopsies in clinical trials. Cancer 119:1357–1364
47. Kim SY, De Vries R, Holloway RG, Kieburtz K (2016) Understanding the 'therapeutic misconception' from the research participant's perspective. J Med Ethics 42(8):522–523
48. Delmonico FL (2009) The implications of Istanbul declaration on organ trafficking and transplant tourism. Curr Opin Organ Transplant 14:116–119
49. Manzano A, Monaghan M, Potrata B, Clayton M (2014) The invisible issue of organ laundering. Transplantation 98:600–603
50. Inglis A, Hippman C, Austin JC (2012) Prenatal testing for Down syndrome: the perspectives of parents of individuals with Down syndrome. Am J Med Genet A 158A:743–745

51. Hill M, Compton C, Karunaratna M, Lewis C, Chitty L (2014) Client views and attitudes to non-invasive prenatal diagnosis for sickle cell disease, thalassaemia and cystic fibrosis. J Genet Couns 23:1012–1021
52. Insogna I, Fiester A (2015) Sterilization as last resort in women with intellectual disabilities: protection or disservice? Am J Obstet Gynecol 212(1):34–36
53. Krumm S, Checchia C, Badura-Lotter G, Kilian R, Becker T (2014) The attitudes of mental health professionals towards patients' desire for children. BMC Med Ethics 15:18
54. Amendola LM, Dorschner MO, Robertson PD, Salama JS, Hart R, Shirts BH, Murray ML, Tokita MJ, Gallego CJ, Kim DS, Bennett JT, Crosslin DR, Ranchalis J, Jones KL, Rosenthal EA, Jarvik ER, Itsara A, Turner EH, Herman DS, Schleit J, Burt A, Jamal SM, Abrudan JL, Johnson AD, Conlin LK, Dulik MC, Santani A, Metterville DR, Kelly M, Foreman AK, Lee K, Taylor KD, Guo X, Crooks K, Kiedrowski LA, Raffel LJ, Gordon O, Machini K, Desnick RJ, Biesecker LG, Lubitz SA, Mulchandani S, Cooper GM, Joffe S, Richards CS, Yang Y, Rotter JI, Rich SS, O'Donnell CJ, Berg JS, Spinner NB, Evans JP, Fullerton SM, Leppig KA, Bennett RL, Bird T, Sybert VP, Grady WM, Tabor HK, Kim JH, Bamshad MJ, Wilfond B, Motulsky AG, Scott CR, Pritchard CC, Walsh TD, Burke W, Raskind WH, Byers P, Hisama FM, Rehm H, Nickerson DA, Jarvik GP (2015) Actionable exomic incidental findings in 6503 participants: challenges of variant classification. Genome Res 25:305–315
55. Bergner AL, Bollinger J, Raraigh KS, Tichnell C, Murray B, Blout CL, Telegrafi AB, James CA (2014) Informed consent for exome sequencing research in families with genetic disease: the emerging issue of incidental findings. Am J Med Genet A 164A:2745–2752
56. McGuire AL, Joffe S, Koenig BA, Biesecker BB, McCullough LB, Blumenthal-Barby JS, Green RC (2013) Ethics and genomic incidental findings. Science 340:1047–1048
57. Viberg J, Hansson MG, Langenskiöld S, Segerdahl P (2014) Incidental findings: the time is not yet ripe for a policy for biobanks. Eur J Hum Genet 22:437–441
58. Wolf SM, Crock BN, Van Ness B, Lawrenz F, Kahn JP, Beskow LM, Cho MK, Christman MF, Green RC, Hall R, Illes J, Keane M, Knoppers BM, Koenig BA, Kohane IS, Leroy B, Maschke KJ, McGeveran W, Ossorio P, Parker LS, Petersen GM, Richardson HS, Scott JA, Terry SF, Wilfond BS, Wolf WA (2012) Managing incidental findings and research results in genomic research involving biobanks and archived data sets. Genet Med 14:361–384
59. Jarvik GP, Amendola LM, Berg JS, Brothers K, Clayton EW, Chung W, Evans BJ, Evans JP, Fullerton SM, Gallego CJ, Garrison NA, Gray SW, Holm IA, Kullo IJ, Lehmann LS, McCarty C, Prows CA, Rehm HL, Sharp RR, Salama J, Sanderson S, Van Driest SL, Williams MS, Wolf SM, Wolf WA, eMERGE Act-ROR Committee and CERC Committee, CSER Act-ROR Working Group, Burke W (2014) Return of genomic results to research participants: the floor, the ceiling, and the choices in between. Am J Hum Genet 94:818–826
60. Jelsig AM, Qvist N, Brusgaard K, Ousager LB (2015) Research participants in NGS studies want to know about incidental findings. Eur J Hum Genet 23:1423–1426
61. Klitzman R, Appelbaum PS, Fyer A, Martinez J, Buquez B, Wynn J, Waldman CR, Phelan J, Parens E, Chung WK (2013) Researchers' views on return of incidental genomic research results: qualitative and quantitative findings. Genet Med 15:888–895
62. Zawati MH, Knoppers BM (2012) International normative perspectives on the return of individual research results and incidental findings in genomic biobanks. Genet Med 14:484–489
63. Wolf SM (2013) Return of results in genomic biobank research: ethics matters. Genet Med 15:157–159
64. Bledsoe MJ, Clayton EW, McGuire AL, Grizzle WE, O'Rourke PP, Zeps N (2013) Return of research results from genomic biobanks: cost matters. Genet Med 15:103–105
65. Cho MK (2008) Understanding incidental findings in the context of genetics and genomics. J Law Med Ethics 36:280–285
66. Van Ness B (2008) Genomic research and incidental findings. J Law Med Ethics 36:292–297
67. Klitzman R, Buquez B, Appelbaum PS, Fyer A, Chung WK (2014) Processes and factors involved in decisions regarding return of incidental genomic findings in research. Genet Med 16:311–317

68. Mathieu G, Groisman IJ, Godard B (2013) Next generation sequencing in psychiatric research: what study participants need to know about research findings. Int J Neuropsychopharmacol 16:2119–2127
69. Appelbaum PS, Roth LH, Lidz CW, Benson P, Winslade W (1987) False hopes and best data: consent to research and the therapeutic misconception. Hast Cent Rep 17:20–24
70. Clayton EW, Ross L (2006) Implications of disclosing individual results of clinical research. JAMA 295:337
71. Townsend A, Adam S, Birch PH, Lohn Z, Rousseau F, Friedman JM (2012) "I want to know what's in Pandora's box": comparing stakeholder perspectives on incidental findings in clinical whole genomic sequencing. Am J Med Genet A 158A:2519–2525
72. Clift KE, Halverson CM, Fiksdal AS, Kumbamu A, Sharp RR, McCormick JB (2015) Patients' views on incidental findings from clinical exome sequencing. Appl Transl Genom 4:38–43
73. Gray SW, Park ER, Najita J, Martins Y, Traeger L, Bair E, Gagne J, Garber J, Jänne PA, Lindeman N, Lowenstein C, Oliver N, Sholl L, Van Allen EM, Wagle N, Wood S, Garraway L, Joffe S (2016) Oncologists' and cancer patients' views on whole-exome sequencing and incidental findings: results from the CanSeq study. Genet Med 18:1011–1019
74. Middleton A, Morley KI, Bragin E, Firth HV, Hurles ME, Wright CF, Parker M, DDD Study (2016) Attitudes of nearly 7000 health professionals, genomic researchers and publics toward the return of incidental results from sequencing research. Eur J Hum Genet 24:21–29
75. Lemke AA, Bick D, Dimmock D, Simpson P, Veith R (2013) Perspectives of clinical genetics professionals toward genome sequencing and incidental findings: a survey study. Clin Genet 84:230–236
76. Strong KA, Zusevics KL, Bick DP, Veith R (2014) Views of nonmedical, health system professionals regarding the return of whole genome sequencing incidental findings. WMJ 113:179–184
77. Rossignol AM, Goodmonson S (1995) Are ethical topics in epidemiology included in the graduate epidemiology curricula? Am J Epidemiol 142:1265–1268
78. Mulhearn TJ, Steele LM, Watts LL, Medeiros KE, Mumford MD, Connelly S (2016) Review of instructional approaches in ethics education. Sci Eng Ethics 23(3):883–912. [Epub ahead of print]
79. Baggerly KA, Coombes KR (2011) What information should be required to support clinical "Omics" publications? Clin Chem 57:688–690
80. Servick K (2015) Can 23andMe have it all? Science 349(1472–1474):1476–1477
81. Roberts JS, Ostergren J (2013) Direct-to-consumer genetic testing and personal genomics services: a review of recent empirical studies. Curr Genet Med Rep 1:182–200
82. Sanfilippo PG, Kearns LS, Wright P, Mackey DA, Hewitt AW (2015) Current landscape of direct-to-consumer genetic testing and its role in ophthalmology: a review. Clin Exp Ophthalmol 43:578–590
83. Zawati MH, Borry P, Howard HC (2011) Closure of population biobanks and direct-to-consumer genetic testing companies. Hum Genet 130:425–432
84. De S, Pietilä AM, Iso-Touru T, Hopia A, Tahvonen R, Vähäkangas K (2019) Information provided to consumers about direct-to-consumer nutrigenetic testing. Public Health Genomics 22:162–173
85. Niemiec E, Howard HC (2016) Ethical issues in consumer genome sequencing: use of consumers' samples and data. Appl Transl Genom 8:23–30
86. Borry P, Howard HC, Sénécal K, Avard D (2010) Health-related direct-to-consumer genetic testing: a review of companies' policies with regard to genetic testing in minors. Familial Cancer 9:51–59
87. Abdul-Karim R et al (2013) Disclosure of incidental findings from next generation sequencing in pediatric research. Pediatrics 131:564–571
88. Shkedi-Rafid S, Dheensa S, Crawford G, Fenwick A, Lucassen A (2014) Defining and managing incidental findings in genetic and genomic practice. J Med Genet 51:715–723

89. Vaught J, Lockhart NC (2012) The evolution of biobanking best practices. Clin Chim Acta 413:1569–1575
90. Jafar TH (2009) Organ trafficking: global solutions for a global problem. Am J Kidney Dis 54:1145–1157
91. Miller CM, Smith ML, Diago Uso T (2012) Living donor liver transplantation: ethical considerations. Mt Sinai J Med 79:214–222
92. Cohen IG (2013) Transplant tourism: the ethics and regulation of international markets for organs. J Law Med Ethic 41:269–285
93. Efrat A (2013) The politics of combating the organ trade: lessons from the Israeli and Pakistani experience. Am J Transplant 13:1650–1654
94. Gill JS, Delmonico FL (2015) Transplant tourism versus proper travel for transplantation. Clin Liver Dis (Hoboken) 6:90–91
95. Sever MS (2006) Living unrelated-commercial-kidney transplantation: when there is no chance to survive. Pediatr Nephrol 21:1352–1356

Chapter 8
Ten Years of Experience in Training Biobank Managers at Master's Level in France

Philip Lawrence, Isabelle Hardy, Elodie Caboux, Jeanne Hélène di Donato, Pierre Hainaut, and Emmanuelle Gormally

Abstract The growing complexity of biobanking requires dedicated professional staff who are literate with the multiple aspects of the biobanking process, including technical, managerial, regulatory, and ethical aspects, and who have a good understanding of the challenges of biospecimen research. Here we describe the structure and achievements of a systematic 2-year training program at the Master's level intended for students with a background in life sciences and providing them with a professional qualification as a "Biobank Manager". This course was initiated in 2010 as a program of the Catholic University of Lyon (France). The multidisciplinary training program includes courses on biobank design and infrastructure, on pre- and post-analytical biospecimen processing, on protocol development, on ethical and regulatory aspects as well as a primer to epidemiology, high-throughput molecular biology, and translational research. In parallel, students also receive generic training in management, budget planning, data analysis, and statistics, as well as 11 months of hands-on internship training in biobanks handling human, animal, plant, or microbial biospecimens. A total of 81 students have graduated since 2012, all of whom found a job within 6 months of graduation.

Keywords Education · Multidisciplinary · Professional activities · Skills · Biobanking science · Management

---

P. Lawrence · I. Hardy · E. Gormally (✉)
Confluence: Sciences et Humanités - UCLy, Lyon, France
e-mail: egormally@univ-catholyon.fr

E. Caboux
International Agency for Research on Cancer, Lyon, France

J. H. di Donato
3CR, Castelginest, France

P. Hainaut
Institute for Advanced Biosciences, INSERM, Université Grenoble Alpes, Grenoble, France

P. Hainaut et al. (eds.), *Biobanking of Human Biospecimens*,
https://doi.org/10.1007/978-3-030-55901-4_8

8.1 Introduction

For the past three decades, developing sample collections for fundamental, applied, and translational research in the public or private sectors has become crucial [1–3]. Technologies, regulations, guidelines, ethics, data and biospecimen management, and quality management systems have evolved to address the challenges of the size and diversity of specimen collections and the multiplication of their usages, leading to a variety of biobank types, structures, and sizes [1, 4–6]. Focusing on biobanks dedicated to research using human samples, a classification for biobanks has been proposed that combines four major elements (type of donor, design, biospecimens, and sponsorship/custodianship) with multiple sub-elements [6]. In terms of organization and management, small biobanks are often managed by small teams (often a single agent) who oversee the entire workflow from specimen collection, processing, storage, and traceability to distribution. In most medium-sized and large biobanks, these tasks are performed by different agents, who may specialize in specific aspects of these activities, ensuring the flow of high-quality biospecimens. In most instances, biobanks are run and staffed by personnel who have formal training in biosciences (biology, medicine, veterinary sciences), often at engineer/technical level, similar to the skills required to support activities in a medical or life sciences laboratory. Whereas this level of education provides adequate training in many practical aspects of biospecimen handling, it does not systematically provide teaching and opportunities for acquiring experience in the type of advanced knowledge required for biobanking, specifically in data management, quality control, ethics, logistic, law and regulations, and management. To address this challenge, we established in 2010 the first graduate program in Europe dedicated to the training of Biobank Managers. In this chapter, we discuss the vision that supports the program, its structure, and its achievements over 10 years of continuous operation and student enrollment.

8.2 Core Activities and Skills of Professional Biobankers

With the development of highly structured biobanks, scientists working in these infrastructures have acquired knowledge and skills not specific to science. Expertise in quality, ethics, law and regulations, and business management are now essential to ensure the maintenance, the development, and the sustainability of biobank infrastructures [7]. Recruiting someone with skills, training, and experience covering this large spectrum might be like looking for a needle in a haystack. Most of the time, this need is addressed by recruiting collaborators that are trained on the job and/or through internal or external courses. Examples of such training programs are listed in Table 8.1. So far, training needs have mostly been addressed by the development of in-house training programs [8], international or national short courses, and by staff exchanges between biobanks. These include courses organized by

Table 8.1 Some examples of Biobank courses available

Title	Organized by	Audience	Objectives	Organization	Duration	Internet address
Introduction to Biobanking Course	Canadian Tumour Repository Network (CTRNet) and the BiobankResource Center	Researchers, biobank staff, stakeholders	Overview of the steps in establishing, maintaining, and using a biobank; Biobank terminology; Principles of optimal human biospecimen handling; Information on standards and practices in biobanks	Online course	15 h	http://www.biobanking.org/brc/webs/education
Principles of Biobanking	University of Luxembourg and Integrated BioBank of Luxembourg (IBBL)	Students, educators, researchers, and practitioners	To provide the theoretical, operational, and practical knowledge needed to run a biobank and to assist in the creation of new biobanks	Lectures, tutorials, visits	3 weeks–90 h	https://wwwfr.uni.lu/formations/fstm/certificate_principles_of_biobanking
Master's in Biobank Management	School in Biology-Biochemistry-Biotechnologies (Catholic University of Lyon, France) in cooperation with Université Claude Bernard Lyon 1	Students, professionnals	Train professionals to coordinate and manage a biobank in a highly international environment	Lectures, laboratory classes, seminars, case studies, visits, biobank internships	2 years	https://www.estbb.fr/en/toutes-nos-formations/biobank-management-graduate/

(continued)

Table 8.1 (continued)

Title	Organized by	Audience	Objectives	Organization	Duration	Internet address
University master's in biobanks and the use of human samples in biomedical research	Catholic University of Valencia (Spain)	Professionals	Provide knowledge for the development of existing or emerging biobanks, their framework in the research system, and their evaluation. Provide knowledge that facilitates the management of biobanks of human samples for research appropriate to the requirements of the regulations	Onsite	1 year	https://www.ucv.es/oferta-academica/posgrados/ciencias-de-la-salud/master-propio-en-biobancos-y-gestion-de-recursos-biologicos-para-investigacion/programa
Msc Biobanking	Medical University of Graz (Austria)	Graduates with a bachelor degree in medicine, technical specialists, and graduates in life sciences	To acquire knowledge, competence, practical skills to work in the multidisciplinary field of biobanking	Blended online/ onsite	2 years	http://postgraduate-school.medunigraz.at/universitaetslehrgaenge/masterlehrgaenge/msc-in-biobanking/

universities such as the 3-week certificate on Biobanking Principles offered by the University of Luxembourg and the Integrated BioBank of Luxembourg (IBBL) [9]. Workshops or online courses on specific biobanking topics are also available. The 3CR (http://www.3cr-ressourcesbiologiques.com/) offers, for example, courses on developing and setting up a quality management system in a biobank. The Biobank Resource Center, a Canadian run initiative, offers an online course called "Introduction to Biobanking" (https://biobanking.org/webs/education/language:brc). The course includes nine modules developed by Canadian scientists and contains country-specific content [10, 11]. However, so far, there has been no general consensus on the development of a comprehensive training roadmap for biobankers, encompassing all aspects of this highly complex activity. Given the rapid expansion of biobanking as a cornerstone activity for research and medicine, it is essential to foster the development of educated professionals who have chosen to develop careers in biobanking, ensuring the growth of a community of specialists who can both fulfill the needs of biobanking in the twenty-first century as well as take up the leadership in the emerging sciences of biospecimens and biobanking [12]. These considerations have led to the construction of a new professional profile for biobank managers, integrating both scientific, managerial and regulatory components into a coherent training and career development path.

The need for professional biobanking is a response to multiple factors and pressures that make it mandatory to develop full mastery of mass preanalytical and analytical workflows. Mastering these workflows, in turn, opens a wealth of opportunities for biotechnologies and biomedicine, in particular, biobanking is a cornerstone for the implementation of "P4 Medicine" (Predictive, Preventive, Personalized, and Participative) and for the interconnection of data from complex analytical processes with data from other sources (connected devices, medical records, health registries, etc.) [13, 14]. Fulfilling this potential requires the identification and development of a set of core biobanking activities, each corresponding to specific skills and knowledge. Table 8.2 lists the core activities and corresponding skills, knowledge, and expertise required for designing, setting up, and running a biobank infrastructure and for ensuring the assembly and accessibility of biospecimens. This list provides an overview of the basic teaching and training needs for professional biobankers encompassing the entire process from designing an infrastructure to running biobanking operations and distributing biospecimen collections.

The biobanking workflow can be described as a pipeline running from biospecimen collection to data integration user, consisting of parallel streams of biological specimen and data flows, embedded in a complex set of ethical, legal, good management, and good laboratory practice regulations, and supporting research aimed at discovery, development, transfer, and value creation. The core activities listed in Table 8.2 are essential at all steps of this pipeline. Even if running this pipeline involves professionals with different backgrounds who will either be supporting or be fully part of the activities of the biobank, it is essential that they all have a precise understanding of the entire biobanking workflow in order to achieve their tasks for the biobank.

Table 8.2 Activities taking place in a biobank and the expertise, skills, and knowledge necessary to conduct them

Activities	Expertise, skills, and knowledge
Biospecimen management	
Organizing and setting up the biobank infrastructure	Biospecimen sciences Health and safety guidelines National and international laws and regulations Preservation and storage methods
Collecting biospecimens	Sources of pre-analytical variability Ethics and bioethics National and international laws and regulations Health and safety guidelines
Supervising pre-analytical treatment of biospecimens	Biospecimen and biomarker sciences Health and safety guidelines
Selecting optimal conservation conditions	Biospecimen and biomarker sciences Storing technologies and cryobiology Protection of biodiversity
Organizing and troubleshooting biospecimen transport	National and international transport regulations Health and safety guidelines
Bringing into service and managing an infrastructure	Quality management system Metrology
Implementing biosafety and biosecurity	Good laboratory practices National and international biosafety and biosecurity regulations
Research and innovation	
Developing and improving collection, pre-analytical, and storing knowledge and protocols	Biospecimen sciences Laboratory management systems
Designing a collection and biobank	Epidemiology, clinical research, environmental science, microbiology, agronomy, veterinary sciences
Involve the biobank in research and innovation	Translational research, veterinary science, agronomy
Characterizing biospecimens Discovering and characterizing biomarkers	Biospecimen and biomarker sciences (analytical biology, biochemistry, chemistry, etc.) Method validation
Implementing research and benchmark strategies for decision-making	Literature review Networking
Data management	
Understanding data structure and selecting appropriate database solutions	Data management Database structure
Selecting Biobank information management systems (BIMS) adapted to biobanking	Knowledge of databases softwares (open sources or commercial) and interoperability
Collecting and storing biospecimen data	Definition of data set requirements Information organization in a database National and international laws and regulations (GDPR) Ethics (confidentiality, data protection) Knowledge of clinical data organization

(continued)

Table 8.2 (continued)

Activities	Expertise, skills, and knowledge
Implementing and ensuring confidentiality	Ethics Data encryption systems National and international laws and regulations (GDPR)
Organizing and implementing traceability of biospecimens and their information	Knowledge of BIMS or LIMS solutions
Extracting and sending appropriate data to biobank users	Data management and interoperability Ethics
Quality management	
Selecting appropriate certification or accreditation	Knowledge of the different types of national and international certification and accreditation (ISO20387, NFS96900, ISO9001)
Setting up the quality management system – Defining the organization and the processes of the biobank – Writing and validating standard operating procedures (SOP) – Maintaining a schedule for the major steps of the SMQ (audits, management review, main actions, and projects) – Preparing and following internal and external quality audits for certification or accreditation	Knowledge of quality assurance, quality control processes
Communicating on the quality management system implemented to collaborators to ensure their understanding of its importance and active compliance	Communication
Ethics	
Identifying and understanding the ethical challenges and taking them into account in everyday work	National and international ethical principles Translate these into everyday practice
Complying to national and international ethical principles	
Documenting the signed informed consent and the ethical clearance	
Protecting the confidentiality of donors and the annonymization of biospecimens	Implement date protection/encryption systems
Consolidating the ethical training and attitude of collaborators	Teaching, training, and educating
Conducting watch on topics related to ethics to implement the latest regulations	Literature survey
Take into account the diversity and complexity of international ethical issues	Awareness of international and intercultural issues
Implementation of laws and regulations	
Implementing national and international laws on human, animal, plant, microorganism biospecimens	Knowledge of legal frameworks
Participating in the setting up of material transfer agreement and contracts for biospecimen transfer to private and public partners	Understand contractualization processes referring to biospecimens

(continued)

Table 8.2 (continued)

Activities	Expertise, skills, and knowledge
Conducting a laws and regulations watch	Litterature review, Networking
Budget management	
Preparing a business plan	Knowledge of budget management and planning Knowledge of principles of accounting
Developing a long-term financial strategy	
Calculating the costs related to biospecimen management	
Establishing a budget according to financial management rules	
Respecting the constraints of a budget, making contingency plans	
Negotiating contracts and equipment costs with suppliers, partners, and users of the biobank	Negotiation
Operational management	
Knowing and implementing the governance of the biobank	Knowledge of organization management principles Knowledge of human resources management Project management Leadership Communication
Knowing and promoting the missions and strategy of the biobank to ensure good governance	
Piloting, planning, managing, anticipating, organizing, coordinating, and driving the activities of a biobank	
Managing, piloting, and completing projects using human, technical, and financial resources to produce deliverables that correspond to the level of quality, cost, and timeframe expected	
Training collaborators to the different activities of the biobank	Knowledge of human resources management Pedagogy
Taking part in the recruitment of collaborators	
Assessing the skills and results of the collaborators	
Organizing and driving a meeting	Organizational management Leadership
Organizing and managing the work of a team	
Developing private/public collaborations	
Taking part in national and international biobank networks	
Communicating orally and in writing about the activities of the biobank using different communication methods	Communication
Conducting a negotiation with multiple parties with different interests keeping in mind the biobank strategic interests	Negotiation Leadership
Risk management	
Developing and implementing a catastrophe prevention and preparedness plan	Knowledge of disaster management Knowledge of risk identification and management
Elaborating a response and recovery strategy	

The diverse and multidisciplinary list of activities and competencies in Table 8.2 identifies an essential aspect of professional biobanking: the professional biobanker operates as a link between different actors, both "upstream" of the biobanking process itself (e.g., the "collectors", scientists or doctors involved in specimen collection) and "downstream" of the process (e.g., the "users", encompassing a large community of laboratory scientists, epidemiologists, and data managers who are exploiting the biobank data and biospecimen resources). Furthermore, the professional biobanker also provides direct support to translational research, by enabling the development of research targeted at improving pre-analytical methods and workflows thus critically contributing to the development and validation of new biomarkers.

8.3 Master's of Biobank Management: A 2-Year Course for Graduates

Since 2010, the School for Biology—Biochemistry—Biotechnologies (ESTBB) at the Catholic University of Lyon (UCLy) has setup a 2-year Master's course in Biobank Management. At the time, this initiative was the first of its kind in France and among the very first worldwide. In Europe, three other Master's courses have been subsequently developed at the Catholic University of Valencia (Spain, 2011), at the Medical University of Graz (Austria, 2016) and at the University of Nice—Sophia Antipolis in France (2016). Since 2011, the Master's course in Valencia has moved to an online course in Spanish whereas the Master's course in Graz blends online and onsite teaching in English.

The Master's course in Lyon is structured as a regular class with onsite, online, and internship components in French. The overreaching goal is to deliver high-level training towards career development in an international environment. It encompasses a broad definition of biobanking, aiming to meet the needs of diverse public and private biobanks, including human, animal, environmental, and microbial biobanks. The course was developed at the initiative of scientists and biobankers, based on the concept that the rapid growth of biobanks and their emergence as major research infrastructure had to be addressed through multidisciplinary training in order to meet academic, societal, and industrial expectations regarding access and usage of high-quality biological resources.

The curriculum of the Master's includes theoretical courses and work experiences in biobanks (Fig. 8.1) that allow students to acquire a total of 120 European Credit Transfer System (ECTS) over 2 years. The basic requirement to register in the Master's is a 3-years Bachelor's Degree in Life Science or equivalent. The theoretical courses are given at ESTBB (Catholic University of Lyon, France) over five periods. The details of the curriculum are described in Table 8.3. Students are offered a number of scientific teaching modules that allow them to specialize in biospecimen sciences and management, as well as providing them with a solid basis

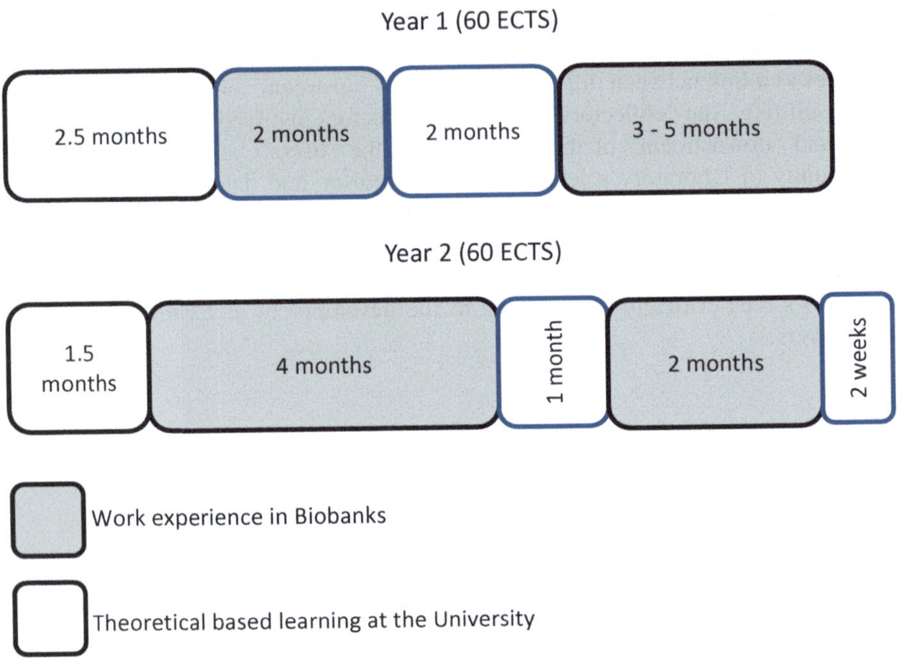

Fig. 8.1 Organization over four semesters of the 2 years Master's "Biobank Management" offered by the Catholic University of Lyon. ECTS: European Credit Transfer System

of essential notions in epidemiology, transfer biomarker research, clinical research, and biostatistics. Training also encompasses management skills (team management, project management, financial management, quality system management, data management). In addition, training covers specific modules for biobanking, including legal, ethical, and regulatory issues as well as knowledge of biobank networks and of the communities of biobank users.

Specific teaching methods are deployed for each module. Training and teaching include lectures, conferences, workshops, laboratory classes, case studies, working groups, site visits to private and public biobanks in the fields of human and animal health and agronomy, as well as extensive work experiences in public or private biobank environments in France or abroad. The course faculty includes over 100 members, including mostly experts in biobanking or biospecimen/biomarker resources (76%) as well as professionals in charge of modules such as management or intercultural communication (10%) and 14% university lecturers in charge of general courses (epidemiology, statistics, health economy, etc.).

In conjunction with their theoretical training modules, students spend time in biobanks through several work experiences (internships) organized in four different periods, providing for a minimum of 11 months of biobanking experience (Fig. 8.1) over the 2-year course. In the first year of the Master's, students are invited to select

Table 8.3 Modules of the Master's Management of Biobanks

Period	Module	Objectives	Teaching method	Duration
Year 1–Semester 1	Biospecimen sciences and biomarkers	List and describe all the biospecimens that can be stored in a biobank Describe the use and analysis of biospecimens	Lectures, laboratory practical, case study, group work, visits	50 h
	Biospecimen management	List and describe the methods for biospecimen collection, pre-analysis, and storage Manage the flow of biospecimens	Lectures, laboratory practical, case studies, group work, visits	36 h
	Biobanks and biobanking: Biobanks storing human biospecimens	Develop and organize a global insight of the different types of biobanks storing human biospecimens	Conferences, bibliography	32 h
	Tools for the work environment and career development	Develop skills essential for an international career in management and science	Workshop, case studies, group work, serious game	59 h
	Work experience in a biobank	Observe and take part in all the activities of a biobank	Work experience, tutorial	4 months
Year 1–Semester 2	Quality management systems	Describe, interpret, and apply the ISO20387, ISO9001, NFS96900, and ISO17025 norms List and analyze the steps to validate methods	Lectures, practicals, case study	33 h
	Data management and databases	List the specifications required for a biobank database Organize the security and traceability of biospecimens and their associated data Communicate on collections	Lectures, exercise class, demonstrations of softwares, visits	40 h
	Biobanks and biobanking: Biobanks storing animal, environmental, microbial biospecimens, natural history museums	Develop and organize a global insight of the different types of biobanks storing nonhuman biospecimens	Conferences, bibliography	29 h
	Tools for the work environment and career development	Develop skills essential for an international career in management and science	Workshop, lectures, personal work, e-learning, tutorials	47 h
	Work experience in a biobank	Develop a project on biobanking in a public or private biobank	Work experience, scientific writing, tutorials	3 months

Table 8.3 (continued)

Period	Module	Objectives	Teaching method	Duration
Year 2–Semester 3	Management, human resources, and financial management	Describe the different methods for team management List and use the different tools available to the manager Describe and use financial accounting tools Describe and analyze a business strategy	Lectures, workshop, exercises, role play	49 h
	Methodologies in clinical research and epidemiology	Describe the methods and protocols of clinical trials Describe the different types of epidemiological studies and their associated methods	Lectures, case study	41 h
	Biobanks and biobanking: Biobank networks	Develop and organize a global insight of expert or biospecimen national and international networks	Conferences, bibliography, group work	22 h
	Tools for the work environment and career development	Develop skills essential for an international career in management and science	Workshop, lectures	44 h
	Work experience in a biobank	Develop a project on biobanking in a public or private biobank	Work experience, scientific writing, and communication, tutorials	4 months
Year 2–Semester 4	Ethics applied to biobanks	Discover and understand ethical principles and apply the knowledge to the context of a biobank Clarify the issues of donation, informed consent, and dignity	Lecturer, tutorials, case study	29 h
	Laws and regulations applied to biobanks	Describe French Laws on individual rights Describe French regulations related to biobanks Describe French regulations related to industrial property Use material transfer agreements for biospecimen cessions	Lecturers, exercise classes	46 h

	Biobanks and biobanking: Private and public users of biobanks	Develop and organize a global insight of the different types of private (small and large companies, nonprofitable organizations such as patient groups) and public (for example, epidemiologists) actors that interact with biobanks to collect or use biospecimens	Conferences, bibliography, and tutorials, visits	25 h
	Tools for the work environment and career development	Develop skills essential for an international career in management and science	Lectures, workshops, personal work	32 h
	Work experience in a biobank	Develop a project on biobanking in a public or private biobank	Work experience, tutorials, master's thesis, viva	2.5 months

two different placements that offer them exposure to a broad range of biobanking experiences (in France or abroad, in a private or in a public biobank, in biobanks managing human, animal, environmental and microbial biospecimens, etc.). The objectives of this first work experience are to get acquainted with the broad spectrum of biobank-related activities and to have the opportunity to participate in or observe a large panel of these activities. Subsequent work experiences (in the second year of the Master's) are focused on the development of a personal project within a biobank, with emphasis on projects that directly pertain to the development, upgrade or quality control of these biobanks (rather than on their routine activities). Projects entrusted to students may include the organization or the management of a new biospecimen collection, the development of new collection, pre-analytical or storage protocols, the writing of specifications for an adapted data management tool, the selection, setting up, and validation of such a tool, the development of a quality management system (QMS), the assessment of ethical and regulatory aspects of the biobank and its compliance with national/international standards, etc. The academic output of the project consists of a Master's thesis, which is presented both in a written report and during a viva examination to a jury consisting of biobanking experts and professors.

Seven groups of students have graduated since 2012 with a total of 81 professionals. These students did their placements in biobanks in France, the UK, Switzerland, Canada, Australia, Ireland, the US, Austria, Luxembourg, Belgium, Sweden, Turkey, Madagascar, and Cambodia. These biobanks belonged to the national public sector (54%), private sector (23.7%), foundations (17.9%), and international organizations (4.4%). Overall, 80% of the students found a job in biobanking immediately after graduation, and 100% were in employment within 6 months of graduating. A total of 31% of them were recruited in the same biobank as where they did their second-year internship. Examples of placements and jobs are presented in Table 8.4.

In addition to students with no prior working experience, the course also welcomes professionals who are already in employment in a biobank. These professionals may follow the entire curriculum or attend specific modules. In addition, the Master's provides for the possibility for professionals with extensive experience in biobanking (minimum 1 year) to pass the graduation on the basis of work experience within the scheme of the French VAE (Validation des Acquis de l'Expérience). VAE is a French program that allows professionals to obtain diplomas by the validation of skills and expertise relevant to the diploma, acquired through their professional or private experience.

Table 8.4 Examples of graduate jobs in public and private biobanks and companies

Job title	Biospecimen	Type of employer
Data manager in virology	Animal	Private company
Sample Flow Manager	Microorganisms	Private company
Biobank platform coordinator	Human	National Biobank
Biobank network coordinator	Human	French regional network
In charge of the valorization of biological resources	Human	Hospital biobank

8.4 Discussion and Perspectives

With the development and professionalization of biobanks, the training of biobank personnel has become critical in fulfilling the scientific, translational, and industrial promises of this rapidly expanding field while complying with the legal, regulatory, and ethical requirements of such infrastructures. Training programs for biobank collaborators have been developed in many places but in most instances, these programs consist of short, ad hoc courses targeted at professionals already engaged in biobanking activities. The objective of the Master's program developed in Lyon is to specifically train postgraduate students as professional biobankers thus supporting the emergence of a curriculum and job definition for individuals who will devote their careers to biobanking and the management of biospecimen resources. Based on 10 years of experience, the multidisciplinary teaching program developed for the Master's course combines in-depth understanding of biospecimen/biomarker sciences, methodological knowledge (epidemiology, statistics, clinical research, and health economy), knowledge and familiarity with legal, regulatory and ethical issues, and development of personal capacities/skills in the management of teams, projects, budgets, and organizations. The success of Master's degree students in finding employment in biobanking organizations after graduating, speaks for the need to develop this curriculum and supports its adaptation to different languages and educational contexts.

Training professional biobankers has become a fundamental need for the sustained development of infrastructures for biological resources. Indeed, over the past 20 years, the field of biobanking has undergone an exponential development and it can be estimated that, within the next decade, several billion biospecimens will be preserved in biobanks around the world. After the wave of creation, biobanks are now facing the challenge of sustainability and continuity [6, 15]. This can be achieved only if biobanks are managed by highly trained, dedicated, and stable staff, who devote their careers to the long-term management and exploitation of biospecimen resources. It also requires that the job title of "Specialist Biobanker" be highly recognized and valued, constituting an appealing career path for young graduates in Life Sciences and related fields. The development of a Master's degree in Biobanking is the cornerstone for raising the profile of these activities and for increasing the awareness of students and the community towards the specific requirements of this activity.

Another essential challenge for the development and sustainability of biobanks is convergence and interoperability through the adoption of international standards (OECD, 2009 (https://www.oecd.org/sti/biotech/44054609.pdf); NCI, 2011 (https://biospecimens.cancer.gov/bestpractices/2011-ncibestpractices.pdf); ISBER, 2012 (http://c.ymcdn.com/sites/www.isber.org/resource/resmgr/Files/ISBER_Best_Practices_3rd_Edi.pdf); IARC, 2017 (http://www.iarc.fr/en/publications/pdfs-online/wrk/wrk2/Standards_ProtocolsBRC.pdf)). The publication by the International Organization for Standardization of the "ISO20387 Biotechnology—Biobanking—General requirements" for biobanks will also play a major role in harmonization [16]. While such standards are being developed and promoted by various national and international bodies [17–20], their implementation requires that a common "biobanking culture" be shared by the main actors in the field, that is, the staff who are in charge of operating biobanks. The development of this Master's course contributes to these objectives by defining the foundations of a common culture and by helping trained biobankers to recognize themselves as a community.

Future steps in education towards biobanking should involve the development of an online curriculum, enabling distance learning and better access to knowledge, in particular, for students from emerging and low-resource countries where biobanking activities will be vital in promoting research fields in the human and animal health, agronomic and environmental challenges facing these countries [21]. Such courses may also include/lead to the development of postgraduate curricula focusing on "biospecimen science," the research area that deals with the development of new methods and knowledge on the acquisition, qualification, and usage of biospecimen resources [22, 23]. Such an advanced curriculum should deliver a degree at PhD level thus supporting a strong dynamic of research in Biobanking and providing further opportunities for personal education and career development for graduates with a Master's degree in Biobanking.

Disclaimer Where authors are identified as personnel of the International Agency for Research on Cancer/World Health Organization (IARC/WHO), the authors alone are responsible for the views expressed in this article and they do not necessarily represent the decisions, policy or views of the International Agency for Research on Cancer/WHO.

References

1. Artene S-A, Ciurea ME, Purcaru SO, Tache DE, Tataranu LG, Lupu M et al (2013) Biobanking in a constantly developing medical world. ScientificWorldJournal 2013:343275
2. Hofman P, Bréchot C, Zatloukal K, Dagher G, Clément B (2014) Public-private relationships in biobanking: a still underestimated key component of open innovation. Virchows Arch Int J Pathol 464(1):3–9
3. Coppola L, Cianflone A, Grimaldi AM, Incoronato M, Bevilacqua P, Messina F et al (2019) Biobanking in health care: evolution and future directions. J Transl Med 17(1):172
4. Shickle D, Griffin M, El-Arifi K (2010) Inter- and intra-biobank networks: classification of biobanks. Pathobiol J Immunopathol Mol Cell Biol. 77(4):181–190
5. Watson PH, Barnes RO (2011) A proposed schema for classifying human research biobanks. Biopreserv Biobank 9(4):327–333
6. Watson PH, Nussbeck SY, Carter C, O'Donoghue S, Cheah S, Matzke LAM et al (2014) A framework for biobank sustainability. Biopreserv Biobank 12(1):60–68
7. Castellanos-Uribe M, Gormally E, Zhou H, Matzke E, Watson P (2020) Biobanking education. Biopreserv Biobank 18(1):1–3
8. Williams RR, Gupta D, Yong WH (2019) Orientation and training of new biobank personnel. Methods Mol Biol 1897:51–63
9. Castellanos-Uribe M, May ST, Betsou F (2020) Integrated biobank of Luxembourg-University of Luxembourg: university biobanking certificate. Biopreserv Biobank 18(1):7–9

10. Matzke EAM, O'Donoghue S, Barnes RO, Daudt H, Cheah S, Suggitt A et al (2012) Certification for biobanks: the program developed by the Canadian tumour repository network (CTRNet). Biopreserv Biobank 10(5):426–432
11. Hartman V, Gali B, Dee S, O'Donoghue S, Tarling T, Barnes R et al (2019) Canadian tissue repository network biobank certification program: update and review of the program from 2011 to 2018. Biopreserv Biobank 17(6):530–538
12. Bornstein SR, Licinio J (2011) Improving the efficacy of translational medicine by optimally integrating health care, academia and industry. Nat Med 17(12):1567–1569
13. Hewitt RE (2011) Biobanking: the foundation of personalized medicine. Curr Opin Oncol 23(1):112–119
14. Vogt H, Hofmann B, Getz L (2016) The new holism: P4 systems medicine and the medicalization of health and life itself. Med Health Care Philos 19(2):307–323
15. De Souza YG (2015) Sustainability of biobanks in the future. Adv Exp Med Biol 864:29–35
16. Tarling T, O'Donoghue S, Barnes R, Carvalho K, Gali B, Castelhano M et al (2020) Comparison and analysis of two internationally recognized biobanking standards. Biopreserv Biobank 18(2):82–89
17. Hewitt R, Hainaut P (2011) Biobanking in a fast moving world: an international perspective. J Natl Cancer Inst Monogr 2011(42):50–51
18. Vaught JB, Caboux E, Hainaut P (2010) International efforts to develop biospecimen best practices. Cancer Epidemiol Biomark Prev 19(4):912–915
19. Henderson MK, Matharoo-Ball B, Schacter B, Kozlakidis Z, Smits E, Törnwall O et al (2017) Global biobank week: toward harmonization in biobanking. Biopreserv Biobank 15(6):491–493
20. Mate S, Kampf M, Rödle W, Kraus S, Proynova R, Silander K et al (2019) Pan-European data harmonization for biobanks in ADOPT BBMRI-ERIC. Appl Clin Inform 10(4):679–692
21. Mendy M, Caboux E, Sylla BS, Dillner J, Chinquee J, Wild C et al (2014) Infrastructure and facilities for human biobanking in low- and middle-income countries: a situation analysis. Pathobiol J Immunopathol Mol Cell Biol 81(5–6):252–260
22. Vaught JB, Henderson MK (2011) Biological sample collection, processing, storage and information management. IARC Sci Publ 163:23–42
23. Ellervik C, Vaught J (2015) Preanalytical variables affecting the integrity of human biospecimens in biobanking. Clin Chem 61(7):914–934

Chapter 9
National Biobank Networking: The Case of Spain

Manuel M. Morente, Francisco Luna-Crespo, Nuria Ajenjo, Maria-Jesus Artiga, and Eva Ortega-Paino

Abstract The last 20 years have been a revolutionary period for biomedical research, mainly because of biotechnological developments that open exciting prospects for a more personalized approach to healthcare with a major impact on prevention, diagnosis, prognosis, and treatment of many human diseases. Biobanks and biobank networks are key pieces in this process, and there are various suitable models and designs.

This chapter presents the progressive development of a nationwide network of biobanks in Spain, and focuses mainly on standardization efforts for technical procedures, ethical requirements, unified quality control policy, and, above all, public service.

Three main stages of this development can be distinguished. The first one (2000–2010) was characterized by early cooperative initiatives to advance cancer research by the Spanish National Cancer Research Centre (CNIO) with a nationwide scope, and by other institutions with a regional focus. These combined efforts allowed the transition from private/institutional collections to true biobanks and biobank networks. The second period (2003–2010) was characterized by a more structured organization following the "network of networks" design in the context of cancer research promoted by cooperating institutions. Finally, since 2010 the Spanish National Biobank Network, founded and funded by the Spanish National Institute of Health Carlos III (ISCIII), has been operative, enlarging its scope to include in 2021 biomodels to become The National Platform for Biobank and Biomodels.

Spanish National Biobank Network is funded with public funds from the Instituto de Salud Carlos III, under the Health Strategic Actions 2010–2013. 2014–2017, and 2018–2020.

M. M. Morente (✉)
Spanish National Cancer Research Centre (CNIO) Biobank, Madrid, Spain

Spanish National Biobank Network, Madrid, Spain

F. Luna-Crespo · N. Ajenjo · M.-J. Artiga · E. Ortega-Paino (✉)
Spanish National Cancer Research Centre (CNIO) Biobank, Madrid, Spain
e-mail: fdeluna@cnio.es; najenjo@cnio.es; mjartiga@cnio.es; eortega@cnio.es

P. Hainaut et al. (eds.), *Biobanking of Human Biospecimens*,
https://doi.org/10.1007/978-3-030-55901-4_9

Keywords Spanish National Biobank Network · Biobanking in Spain · Biobank networking · Biobank cooperation · Biobanking

9.1 Biobank Networking is the Challenge for Biobanking in the Twenty-First Century

The last decade of the twentieth century was the scene of a biotechnological revolution in the developed world. It was characterized not only by new methods for genomic and proteomic studies but also by the ability to transfer this technology effectively and efficiently to many research areas and to the clinical setting ("from bench to bedside"). These technical developments renewed interest in "translational research": a real translation of recently acquired basic biomedical knowledge into the promotion of health, with the medium/long-term challenge of a more personalized medicine. This biotechnological, investigative, and clinical revolution needs to be built from high-quality tissue samples and associated data, otherwise, the use of low-quality samples and poorly documented associated information will surely lead to erroneous results and invalid conclusions [1, 2]. In addition, the size of research studies has increased dramatically, and the focus of current biomedical research is now different. Present studies focus on:

- **Identification of new parameters of clinical value**, which demands large-scale molecular studies from large numbers of cases.
- **Transfer of knowledge from basic to clinical research**, which requires homogeneous tissue-sampling protocols for multicenter studies.
- **Validation of results obtained in animal models and human cell lines**, which requires providing clinically relevant human samples to basic research groups.
- **Prediction of treatment response**, based on clinical trials including the acquisition of suitable clinical samples for molecular studies.

Today's biomedical research of excellence is a global phenomenon, organized mainly around the study of large series of samples, including specific patient information, following well-defined and detailed criteria.

Translational research is a bidirectional movement between basic and clinical research. Biobanks are precisely at the crossroads of this movement, allowing basic and applied researchers to use high-quality tissues and data, according to their needs. Easy access to high-quality biological samples and their associated data is, currently, the main bottleneck for the development of biomedical research, and biobanks are the main tool to prevent this bottleneck. For this purpose, biobanks need to be considered not as mere storage or repository locations with information recorded on a spreadsheet, but rather as recognized institutions responsible for managing all the required procedures and resources for suitable biospecimen management. They must have an intensive and creditable quality control policy and be generally (but not always) integrated into the clinical activity, given that human samples are very special by themselves, often very difficult to obtain and subject to a specific and strict ethical and legal framework.

To face these challenges, various suitable models and designs have been developed: isolated banks or cooperative networks, prospective and/or retrospective collections, project or non-project driven, monographic or generic, private or public, commercial or nonprofit, local vs regional vs national vs international networks, etc. [3–6]. All these models may be useful or not, depending on how they respond to market needs, and knowledge of these needs is best obtained through a thorough stakeholders' analysis of stakeholders' needs. Specific goals require specific designs, and the best practices for banking depend on the repository goals [7].

It can be stated that human sample collections have always been there since pathology departments have always stored tissue sample blocks [1, 8] and these have been used not only for diagnosis but also for important research activities. However, due to the abovementioned present-day scientific challenges, the current biobank definition has evolved in order to provide a better service in translational research, including harmonization of network-associated biorepositories. They allow access to high quality samples to both applied and basic researchers in a context that safeguards the donor's rights and the quality of the research [9].

But not only biobanks are obliged to move forward to a more appropriate design, networking in terms of public service is absolutely essential in order to fulfill current scientific requirements [5, 10] since it is a cornerstone in the knowledge-based bioeconomy [11, 12].

9.2 The Spanish Route from Private/Institutional Collections to True Biobanks and Biobank Networks

In Spain, as in most scientifically developed countries, a large number of private or public research institutions need biorepositories or collections of human samples. In fact, most of the currently accepted clinical entities were defined in the twentieth century by a clinical-pathological approach based on the study of samples collected through collaborations between clinicians and pathologists. Almost every translational investigation in Spain has been done in the hospital setting. In parallel, and almost without effective connections with the clinical activity, basic researchers produced a plethora of data, focusing on the basic mechanisms of the disease using mostly cell lines and animal models. The tissue sample collections were generally only used by individual researchers and/or institutional research centers lacking a public service view.

In order to respond to the new scientific requirements, and based on the original design of some national and regional initiatives, a biobank networking activity arose in the year 2000 in Spain, mainly oriented to cancer research. These activities share common views regarding what tumor banking is supposed to involve in the twenty-first century, including:

- Not just a tissue storage service but also a series of hospital protocols that allow molecular studies of tumor samples.
- Collection, freezing, and storage of neoplastic and normal tissues ought to be considered a routine practice in the pathology and hematology departments.
- Biobanking is not only a pathologist's activity, but a global hospital responsibility involving surgeons, oncologists, hematologists, hospital managers, and, obviously, pathologists.
- Homogeneous and suitable protocols for the collection, handling, storage, and use of samples for research, teaching, and cancer patient care.
- Being open to sharing tissue samples with basic and applied researchers.
- More specialized dedication of the personnel directly working in these units.
- Strict ethical protocols guaranteeing the rights of the patients and society.
- Quality assurance and quality control practices under a comprehensive quality management system.

The earliest of these initiatives was initiated by the Spanish National Cancer Research Centre (CNIO) in September 2000. The Spanish National Tumor Bank Network was created and coordinated by the CNIO's Molecular Pathology Program, and aimed to satisfy the demand for human neoplastic tissue under ideal conditions for the development of large-scale studies of clinical significance in Spain, and for small size high-quality series for basic researchers.

As a national center, the first goal of this initiative was to promote high-quality tumor banks within every Spanish hospital, as a public service. Next, these banks were invited to participate in a collaborative network: The Spanish National Tumor Bank Network. Although its design corresponded to a hospital-based decentralized network, the activity relied strongly on a central coordination office (CNIO) that assumed leadership following the so-called honest broker role [13] and that guaranteed confidentiality, stability, QA/QC policy, homogeneous protocols, and recognition by research agencies and ethical review boards.

The Spanish National Tumor Bank Network finished its activities in 2010 due to the natural development of hospital-based biobanks, according to the specific effective legislation. During its 5 last years of life (from 2006 to 2010), the network facilitated and participated in 233 scientific projects, most of them from multicenter cooperative groups, corresponding to 505 requests for tissue and data. The median impact factor of the 96 supported publications where the source of samples and data were explicitly cited was 6.355. We also provided samples and/or registry and tracking support to the CNIO Human Cancer Genetics Program (454 familial cancer cases), and directly participated in 29 collaborative projects and clinical trials. But more relevant than these figures is probably the fact that this Network was the first open collaborative experience of a nationwide biobank network in the world, demonstrating that such an innovative challenge was possible and could be successful.

9.3 Spanish Tumor Bank Network of Networks

Following this design, new networks arose in parallel from 2001 to 2005 in four Spanish autonomous regions: Castile and Leon, Catalonia, Asturias, and Andalusia. All these networks were based on overtly collaborative structures. This regional development must be understood in the context of the Spanish National Healthcare Sytem design. From the political and administrative point of view, Spain is divided into 17 autonomous regions (Autonomous Communities) with decentralized specific responsibilities including healthcare, which mainly belongs to the public sector.

The existence of four regional biobank networks and one network with a nationwide scope, far from being a problem, was a great platform for national collaboration based on a common basic design. Independent of the network in which they are included, sample collections stay in their original institution, where they can be used for clinical diagnosis, teaching, and research activities, and the institution is the only one responsible for its own biobank activity. However, if a multicenter project requires samples from different institutions, different biobanks coordinate themselves through a coordination node and are able to respond efficiently to the query; they all apply the same standards, defined by the implementation of common SOPs. This generally accepted network model does not correspond to a central biobank, but to a cooperative and coordinated network of hospital banks, based on homogeneous and optimal tissue-treatment protocols, and interconnected by a computer-based network (LIMS).

Each network had a central coordination office that guaranteed confidentiality, stability, QA/QC policy, homogeneous protocols, recognition by research agencies and ethical review boards, and leadership, following the so-called honest broker role. This design has three layers of activity: hospital-based, regionally promoted and managed, and centrally coordinated.

From 2003, this collaboration became more effective through the Thematic Network of Cooperative Research of Cancer Centers (RTICCC) promoted by the Instituto de Salud Carlos III (Spanish Ministry of Health), which included a specific tumor banking activity with the involvement of 23 hospital tumor banks, most of them associated with either regional or the abovementioned National Tumor Bank Network promoted by the CNIO.

During 2003 and 2004, the early RTICCC period, the Tumor Bank program created a suitable framework of networking and harmonization to use the same technical protocols, the same homogeneous ethical requirements, a unique sample identification system, and a common quality control program. All of these issues were agreed upon by consensus.

The development of the RTICCC-Tumour Banking Programme was based on the confluence of the regional and supra-regional initiatives mentioned above and on the organization and financial support by the RTICCC, which in turn was based on: (a) development of regional networks; (b) uniformity in the organization model, methodologies, and ethical-legal fundamentals; and (c) the development of a quality control/quality assurance policy. The first two initiatives were started along with the program, while the third started during the third year of the program in order to test the quality of some aspects of it.

Once the RTICCC Tumor Bank Programme had started, every local tumor bank coordinator was invited to join working groups for the elaboration of consensus documents, as well as to start an informative and supportive campaign aimed at the regional health agencies. Moreover, this campaign provided anurge for the creation of well-developed regional networks.

A coordination role was assigned to the CNIO and two main centers: Cancer Research Center (CIC) in Salamanca and Clinic-IDIBAPS Hospital in Barcelona. This decision was based on two main reasons: first, cancer research in Spain is concentrated in monographic centers in Madrid, Barcelona, and Salamanca; and secondly, the CNIO provides the experience and the foundations in tumor bank networking.

The achievement of similar organizational structures in each region, coupled with standardized protocols for the handling, storage, and sharing of samples was considered of major importance for the success of the program, and, therefore, for future stable supra-regional biobank network. Thus, a consensus document dealing with organization, methodology, database design and management, and ethical-legal issues was elaborated with the involvement of all local coordinators from the RTICCC tissue banks.

Briefly, an organization scheme was proposed that consisted of a net of regional biobank networks, each one with a coordination node in charge of managing requests to the regional network and a central regional database. Methodology requirements dealt with the time of ischemia, selection-freezing-storage processes and shipment according to international guidelines [14, 15]. Indications and requirements regarding the design of databases capable of complying with the current legislation and necessary interconnections with other regions, as well as a central national database, were also included in the consensus documents.

The quality policy was conceived to involve all aspects of tumor banking including procurement, preservation, shipment, data management, and ethical-legal aspects, not only in the local tumor bank but also in the regional/national network as well. Every bank was in charge of defining its own quality requirements according to their capabilities. Yet, a minimum of quality requirements was established in the consensus document. For instance: less than half an hour of ischemia time, selection of samples performed by a pathologist (or trainee), storage at −80 °C or lower, freezer alarms and back-up freezer space, informed consent, reviews carried out by an ethics committee, etc.

A quality control survey was designed and conducted in 2005 to test several randomly chosen samples of each bank for morphological, immunohistochemical (antigenic preservation of CD31, vimentin, and MIB1 expression on a tissue microarray with all samples), and molecular quality (integrity of mRNA tested using an Agilent Bioanalyzer®). This first survey yielded very encouraging results, given the good morphological, immunophenotypical, and molecular properties of the samples in most instances. Samples yielded good quality RNA in 97% of cases. The immunohistochemical results on paraffin-embedded tissues showed that samples were processed and selected in an adequate manner, although there was a slight variability with respect to MIB1 expression. In particular, there were a few samples (4%) in which the expression of this epitope was either very weak or negative in tumor cells, suggesting the effect of a long fixation period of the samples used for the analysis. We therefore recommended each tumor bank to obtain specific paraffin blocks, whenever possible, with a very controlled fixation time. According to the experience of several members of the network, this is very important for tissue microarray studies.

The main activity of the RETICC Tumor Bank Program occurred during the period 2003–2006 [16]. The Network of Cooperative Research of Cancer Centers continued its research activities, but a transcendental event transformed the whole Spanish biobank activity in 2007 when a new Act on Biomedical research was approved by the Spanish Parliament. This act included, for the first time, general rules for biobanking. These rules were developed further in a Royal Decree in December 2011 [17, 18]. In addition, the promotion of a comprehensive Biobank Network (see below) made the Tumor Bank Program less necessary, and its activities were transferred to a wider initiative: The Spanish National Biobank Network.

9.4 The Spanish National Biobank Network (2010–2013)

In 2009, the Spanish National Institute of Health Carlos III (ISCIII), funding agency of the Ministry of Science and Innovation, through its call for grants of the Strategic Action in Health 2010–2013, decided to promote a National Biobank Network in order to add value to the Spanish biobank system under the recent Biomedical Research Act, and to provide an appropriate service platform to be integrated into the pan-European infrastructure of biobanking, Biobanking and Biomolecular Resources Research Infrastructure (BBMRI-ERIC) [19].

This initiative of the ISCIII aimed at consolidating and recognizing the cooperative efforts regarding hospital-based biobanks developed in our country over the last decade, and made a greater degree of integration, harmonization, and public service possible thus adding value to the whole Spanish Biobank System.

The Network initially integrated 63 institutions from 15 of the 17 Spanish Autonomous Regions. These institutions were selected through a competitive process and included 52 hospital biobanks associated with the National Health System and 11 other institutions, such as the National DNA Bank, research institutions, private hospitals, and several coordination centers of regional biobank networks. Every center was evaluated once per year, and the funds allocated to them depended on compliance with local and cooperative commitments.

The Network was meant to be a meeting point for these biobanks to increase the quality and homogeneity of the services they provided, and to facilitate access to biological samples of human origin and their associated data by the National Health

System (NHS) as a whole with the best quality standards and the assurance that donor rights would be respected according to the existing legal framework.

The Spanish Biobank Network was established as a stable biobank network for biomedical research with five main characteristics:

- Essentially, but not exclusively, hospital-based and disease-oriented.
- With a clear vision dedicated to public service.
- Committed to applicable ethical principles and with a strict observance of the domestic and European legislation in force.
- Based on maximum respect for regional and territorial initiatives and/or initiatives taken by every center.
- The network was organized and structured to function as a stable instrument of coordination among its members.

The Spanish National Biobank Network focused on developing a cooperative public service platform made up of hospital biobanks, regional network platforms of associated biobanks, and other institutions with activities related to sample management that is especially directed at the Spanish scientific community to meet the following challenges:

- To provide access to quality sample collections and associated data to the scientific community through a cooperative structure of public service, mostly implemented in hospitals.
- To integrate existing biobanking initiatives establishing a functional roadmap of biobanks.
- To promote the creation of varied high-quality collections, fitting current needs of researchers and those that can be foreseen for the future (fit for purpose).
- To harmonize their functional strategies, technical processes, and procedures in line with the ethical and legal requirements.
- To ensure respect of the fundamental rights and free will of patients and donors, with special reference to the protection of individual dignity and identity, from which the principle of autonomy derives, and of the treatment of their personal data.
- To promote technological innovation in biobanks.
- To assist in the development of the pan-European platform BBMRI-ERIC, and to promote Spanish participation in the infrastructure.

Summarizing the **mission** of the cooperative infrastructure, the Biobank Network aimed to provide the Spanish biobank system with added value by creating a harmonious cooperative framework for the benefit of the Scientific Community, favoring the growth of scientific production in biomedicine both in quantity and especially in quality, while guaranteeing the patient's rights with respect to donation, management, and transfer of biological samples and associated information within the framework of ethical and legal standards.

The Network activity does not compete with the responsibilities of the Health Authorities or the institutions that host the biobanks, but rather complements their actions, in an open and efficient cooperative framework, through the implementation of harmonized protocols regarding procurement, processing, and sample storage, as well as the collection of clinical data by applying diagnostic criteria and pathology stages, in line with international standards, so as to optimize the quality of the samples and to minimize individual differences inherent to every biobank.

The **vision** of the network includes:

- Be a public service of the highest quality in its field of activities.
- Be a cooperative national reference for biobanks through harmonization of procedures, institutional integration, and organization as a public service for samples and associated data within the framework of Act 14/2007 on Biomedical Research.
- Be designed to have a territorial and functional structure of a "network of networks," similar to the one established in the preliminary design of the European network of biobanks BBMRI (Biobanking and Biomolecular Resources Research Infrastructure).
- Show a strong commitment to its own ethical principles, with a strict observance of the effective legislation.

The **strategic plan** for the period 2010–2013 was developed around three priority axes: Integration, harmonization, and public service.

Integration should be understood as the dynamics of progressive functional integration of all its components into cooperative structures. Within this axis five levels of integration with different strategic objectives were considered:

1. Intra-hospital integration, including:

    (a) To promote the concept that hospital biobanks become the basic tool for managing biological samples and associated data for biomedical research.
    (b) To promote the integration of project-driven collections of biological samples for research into the biobank.
    (c) To improve sample handling circuits in the healthcare system and to promote the organization of the pathology archives and other diagnostic archives as biobanks following the recently published norms while preserving the healthcare needs of patients.
    (d) To promote the implementation of the Biomedical Research Act and its development in a specific biobanking regulatory norm.

2. Integration at the level of the Autonomous Communities, i.e., to collaborate with the regional authorities in the promotion of regional cooperative biobank structures.
3. Integration at the national level, which was in fact the main scope of the network, so as to implement the operational integration of the various biobanks and biobanking networks as nodes of a collaborative matrix structure.
4. International integration, including promoting the participation of the Network and its members in international initiatives and especially in BBMRI-ERIC; this

was at that time classified as a top priority in the Spanish Ministry of Science and Innovation task list.

5. Thematic integration of specific areas, such as brain banks, banks for rare diseases, and neurodegenerative diseases.

Harmonization referred to the development, refinement, and implementation of common standard operating procedures (SOPs) as part of a global network quality policy, including:

1. Harmonization at the technical level SOPs.
2. Harmonization at the legal level, understood as harmonization of criteria arising from the ethical and legal requirements of current applicable legal framework.
3. Quality assurance policies focused on harmonizing and increasing the degree of implementation of quality control procedures in every associated hospital-based biobank.

Public service, an essential part of the Spanish Biobank Network concept, should be understood here both in the internal dimension of the Network itself and in its relationship with the Scientific Community, including researchers and Biobank professionals, health authorities and agencies, without losing sight of patients, donors, and Society as a whole. Thus, this public service was aimed at three levels:

1. The biobanks themselves:
   (a) To enhance and standardize the quality of the biological products and their associated information in the context of the definition given by the OECD of Biological Resource Centers (BRC) [20].
   (b) To promote learning activities, including activities at the highest academic level, that allow the professionalization of the different actors involved in the biobanking activity and to facilitate the harmonization of the terms described above.
   (c) To provide a scientific environment of cooperation and research specifically focused on the biobank activity (biospecimen research).
   (d) To provide advice on the formation of high-quality biobanks.

2. The Scientific Community:
   (a) To provide researchers with a channel that allows quick access to comprehensive sets of samples, their end-products, and the associated data with quality assurance and conforming to ethical-legal regulations.
   (b) To develop a continuous and dynamic analysis and assessment of the needs of biobank end-users.

3. Society: To make biobank activity known to and appreciated by the public, with special attention to patient associations and people suffering from different conditions.

An essential actor in any network in terms of service was at the time a well-organized **coordination office** [10]. Its main functions were to support the scientific coordination and to monitor compliance with the network's objectives set out through its working groups and programmed activities. Its responsibilities also included:

- Strengthen and coordinate network working groups and initiatives of the whole network.
- Implement and coordinate internal policies for quality assurance in the network.
- Create and maintain a management system of biological samples and associated data stored in member biobanks to facilitate their access by the Scientific Community.
- Permanent advisory activity on ethical and legal aspects related to biobanking activities. When needed, this activity was supported by the Bioethics Committee of the Health Institute Carlos III as network external advisors.
- Organize staff training activities to achieve a progressive professionalization of the biobanking activity in hospitals and nodes.
- Joint activities with patient associations and social media to share information about the importance of biobanks for translational research.
- Promote joint activities with domestic and international Scientific Societies and Cooperative Groups.
- Cooperation with other Biobanks that are or could be promoted by the Health Institute Carlos III.
- Official scientific representation in international biobank platforms, especially at the European level.
- Cooperation with health authorities in charge of licensing and maintenance of biobanks, both at the regional and the national level.
- Create and maintain the network website (www.redbiobancos.es) in order to make the Network activities, its objectives, and services known to the scientific community, and to serve as a means of communication between its members and researchers.
- Preparation of monographs and technical documents and bringing together the results of the working groups.

The main operative body of the network in this period was an **Executive Committee**. Made up of 15 members, it was appointed by the National Institute of Health board of directors at the proposal of the Coordinator, according to: operational criteria, training, representation of the different scientific and territorial areas in the network, and expertise. Its functions were to collaborate in the tasks of the coordinator in the various areas of cooperation among network centers, as well as in the tasks of monitoring and fulfilling the action plan approved by ISCIII. This committee assumed the functions of the Interim Scientific Committee.

An **Ethics Advisory Committee** was also implemented to assess the needs regarding biobanking activity, with the aims of protecting the fundamental rights of individuals and respecting the bioethical principles stated in the Convention on Human Rights and Biomedicine [21] and commitments made by the scientific community. This function was assumed by the Research Ethics and Animal Welfare Committee of the ISCIII.

In order to develop all operative aspects of the network, a number of **Working Groups** were created, choosing network members according to their individual and institutional expertise. The fundamental objectives of these working groups were to explore in detail different strategic aspects concerning biobanking and networking activities. Approved by the General Coordinator after consultation with the Executive Board, several working groups took form, some dedicated to horizontal/thematic actions and some that followed transversal/specific action lines; the latter meant to be temporal projects, whereas the first were meant to be permanent, exploring common aspects of the biobanking field. This division allowed the Network to evolve and adapt easily to every aspect of this complex field. Every working group had a coordinator who was automatically included in the Executive Board.

Four thematic and six transversal working groups were created from 2010 to 2013:

1. Thematic working groups (2010–2013):
   (a) Oncological diseases biobanking (coordinator: E. De Alava, Salamanca).
   (b) Biobanking of blood derivatives (M.A. Muñoz, Madrid).
   (c) Brain tissue biobanking (I. Ferrer, Barcelona).
   (d) DNA/population biobanking (A. Orfao, Salamanca).

2. Transversal working groups (2010–2013):
   (a) Best practices guidelines (I. Novoa, Barcelona).
   (b) Informed consent (V. Cusí, Barcelona).
   (c) Quality management policies (A. Garcia-Montero, Salamanca).
   (d) Spanish legal framework for biobanking (R. Bilbao, Bilbao).
   (e) Sustainability and cost analysis of biobanks (O. Fernandez, Santiago de Compostela) [22].
   (f) Applicability of SNOMED-CT to biobank activity (J. Martinez, Valencia).

More than 150 people participated in the working groups from the 63 network members and from organizations outside the network.

Education and training should be a priority action in every biobank network, scientific society, and international platform. There is an urgent need for a new generation of "biobankers" comprehensively trained in all aspects of the complex activity of biobanking. They are needed to take on the development of biobanking in the short and medium term. Between 2010 and 2013, the Spanish Biobank Network developed several initiatives, including monographic short courses and meetings, local lectures, recommended papers on the web, and four annual congresses held in Bilbao (2010), Tarragona (2011), Granada (2012, Joint Meeting with the European, Middle East and Africa society for Biopreservation and Biobanking—ESBB), and Madrid (2013). A special mention is reserved to the most comprehensive and demanding training activity promoted by the Spanish National Biobank Network: a university master's degree organized as a joint activity with the Catholic University of Valencia. Three editions have been completed (2011–2012, 2012–2013, and

2014–2015) with more than 50 graduates. As this chapter is being written, a fourth edition was finished with a completely online format, as a way to expand this experience to Latin-Americans and other Spanish speaker colleagues.

Another key tool for networking is interoperability, to be able to share actionable and comprehensible datasets in a secure framework. For this purpose, an IT platform for interoperability was specifically developed in order to share two types of information: global minimum data sets and project-driven specific minimum data sets. The IT platform is divided according to type of biobank (brain banks, solid tissue banks, population cohorts, etc.) and according to conditions (rare diseases, neurodegenerative diseases, cancer, etc.). The platform was built on SNOMED-CT-based ontology and archetypes, including SPREC (standard pre-analytical coding) and the BRISQ minimum data set integrated [23, 24].

In December 2011, a new Royal Decree (RD1716/2011), that further developed the biomedical research act was approved [17, 18]. It regulates biobanking activities and biobank authorizations in Spain, completing the entire Spanish legal framework in force regarding our activity. This decree is quite complex from the administrative point of view and imposed an obligation on biobanks to be authorized by their corresponding regional bodies. In response to this new legal situation, most of our activities in 2012 were oriented at promoting and integrating the new legal framework into our routines and to assisting our members with its implementation. As an example, this task caused us to organize more than 20 monographic meetings all around the country, including meetings with patient organizations.

At the end of this first funded period, the global balance was very positive. The network was able to promote the Spanish biobank system as a tool that provides an efficient public service and placed the network activities in an international context. However, many issues still remained to be solved.

The main achievements of the National Biobank Network from 2010 to 2013 include:

- Improvement of biobank integration.
- Improvement of local infrastructures.
- High participation in working groups.
- Normalized SOPs and best practices.
- Incorporation of international standards (SNOMED-CT, SPREC, BRISQ).
- IT platform for interoperability.
- Assumption of the new specific legal framework.
- Training.
- Internationalization.

In summary, we laid the foundations for an efficient and robust platform of services. However, it was a road paved with difficulties, especially when trying to persuade about the classic notion best described as the "my syndrome" [25] characterized by isolated resaerch collections and biobanks created exclusively to carry out "my" projects, in contrast to the new conception of biobanking as a public service based on open and friendly cooperation.

9.5 The Spanish National Biobank Network 2014–2017

By June 2013, the Instituto de Salud Carlos III (ISCIII) decided to continue its support to this cooperative initiative in biobanking. This time however a change of model was proposed for the period 2014–2017 which involved moving from a network to a more operative concept of a service platform. The new call once again was competitive, but this time it was based on previously structured platform proposals. This differed from the previous call (2009), which was center-based.

The Executive Committee of the Spanish National Biobank Network assumed the responsibility to elaborate an initial strategic plan and to try to incorporate as many high-quality biobanks as possible, with the objective to present a robust and winning candidacy. The strategic plan was to be more inclusive than selective, and feasible under the announced budget reduction.

The proposed pillars of the new Platform were:

- Consolidate the Spanish biobank system.
- Develop ambitious, evaluable, and feasible objectives.
- Combine the criteria mentioned above with a drastic reduction in funding (less than 50% of the budget during the previous period).
- Fill the need for incorporation of new institutions of excellence.
- Complete selection of the best-associated biobanks from the previous stage.
- Funds allocation needed to be oriented towards promoting the coordination of Spanish biobanks, and their effective integration into a strategic platform of excellence. Equipment will not be funded.

Finally, the proposal was presented, selected, and accepted with a global budget of three million Euros per year for 4 years. However, the platform was subjected to fiscal evaluation every year and the budget may decrease depending on the national economic situation and other unforeseen priorities and circumstances. In fact, during the previous period the budget was reduced up to 50% from 2010 to 2013 due to the national and international economic crisis.

Currently, the network (platform) is composed of 52 institutions, including hospital-based biobanks, research center biobanks, complex biomedical research institutions (hospitals + universities), and regional or thematic biobank networks [26]. Associated institutions (not funded) will be welcomed and promoted.

The current network design is based on five programs:

1. Strategic collections promotion.
2. Networking services.
3. Research & Developmet and innovation (R&D + i) in biobanking.
4. Ethical, legal, and societal issues (ELSI).
5. Coordination, including training and dissemination.

Program 1 Strategic Collections Promotion (Coordinator A. Orfao, Salamanca)
The main objective of this program was to select, build, and offer a catalog of biological samples with associated clinical and/or basic epidemiological information to research projects. It centered its activity on three chapters: population studies, rare diseases, and prevalent disorders affecting adults or children. To deal with these objectives four working groups were created:

1. Population collections: in charge of the promotion of a large cohort representative of the Spanish population, including basic epidemiological data. Three special sub-cohorts will be established corresponding to aged people (>90 years old), twins, and familial triplets (father/mother/one or more sons or daughters).
2. Cohorts of prevalent diseases associated with their corresponding controls. Ten specific working areas were established: cancer and cardiovascular, neurodegenerative, respiratory, digestive, metabolic, renal, ophthalmic, inflammatory, and infectious diseases. Several diagnostic groups (entities) will be established in these areas, mainly in cancer (i.e., breast, colon, upper respiratory tract, lung, leukemia, lymphoma, and others).
3. Rare diseases with special focus on those of special interest and scientific activity in the domestic and international context.
4. Prevalent childhood diseases, including pediatric cancer, genetic and inherited diseases, obesity, etc.

Program 2 Improvement of Networking Services (Coordinator: Ana I. Sáez, Granada)
The central aim of this program was to improve, develop, and implement a global management system to attend better to the requests for samples and data from biomedical researchers, all of which were under a well-established network common quality management policy. Special interest and efforts was oriented towards:

- Providing professionalized attention to researchers with their service requests.
- Elaborating and publishing a catalog of resources including not only samples and data, but also technical infrastructures and facilities.
- Elaborating and publishing a comprehensive services portfolio for researchers.
- Improving a global quality management system complementary to the policies of each associated institution.

Program 3 Research, Development, and Innovation (R&D + i) in Biobanking (Coordinator: Roberto Bilbao, Bilbao)
R&D + i is considered a key component of every biobank. As a network, research and development is essential, and it is the only way to adapt to changes efficiently and to be competitive; in an environment where processes and client needs change all the time, it makes a difference. To obtain better integration, communication, and management systems oriented towards samples and data to establish and improve evidence-based standardized procedures, five initial strategic lines were established:

1. Innovative evidence-based processes and quality markers for blood and cellular derivatives.
2. Innovative evidence-based processes and quality markers for serum and plasma samples.
3. Innovative evidence-based processes and quality markers for solid tissue samples.
4. Data harmonization and adaptation of the biobanking activity to SNOMED-CT.
5. Development of an image-based locator system for banked solid samples.

Program 4 Ethical, Legal, and Social Issues: ELSI (Coordinator: Manuel M Morente, Madrid)
Biobanks should be located between patients/donors, society, and researchers, be a cornerstone and promoter of responsible research. It is in this context that this program needs to be understood: a service to donors and researchers while fulfilling legal requirements. This current program had a clear transversal vocation, and three main strategic lines were developed:

1. Ethical issues: Promoting an ethics observatory for every action included in the previous programs and implementing by consensus, abbreviated procedures for the Ethics Committees associated to biobanks. Also, dissemination of new advances and discussions in biobanking-related ethical issues.
2. Legal issues: Promoting a legal observatory for every action included in the previous programs.
3. Social issues: Focusing on biobank activity and its value for the civil society with special emphasis on patient associations and scientific societies.

Program 5 Coordination, Training, and Communication (Coordinator: Manuel M Morente, Madrid)
The basic competence of this program was to be in charge of the management and to monitor the compliance with the objectives of the platform's programs and the activities of the working groups. Coordination also officially represents the platform. Therefore, it is a purely transversal program and its actions included:

1. Coordination: Global management, promotion, and monitoring of the whole network's activity; authorization of expenditures related to equipment for general use, supplies, and services; presidency of governance bodies (Executive Committee, Steering Committee, and General Assembly); official network representation.
2. Training: Coordination and promotion of regular training activities including an annual meeting and any other training activities required for the remainder of the programs.
3. Internationalization: Promoting an effective participation of the network and its members in international initiatives and institutions. Unfortunately, Spain didnot join BBMRI-ERIC.
4. Dissemination: being in charge of the promotion and permanent updating of the usual channels of dissemination including website, newsletters, publications, social media.

9.6 The Spanish National Biobank Network 2017–2020

In April 2017, the ISCIII approved the competitive call for "support platforms on science and health technologies." Very similar to the previous call, it was based on the presentation of a common scientific proposal supported by the historical records of the units. Each unit (biobank) adhered to a series of projects. Resources were limited, so the ISCIII (as promoter) selected the biobanks that offer value to the overall project.

On this occasion, due to the former direction retirement, the board elected among their members an interim coordinator (Cristina Villena, PhD, from CIBERESP pulmonary biobank) in order to lead the design of the project and modified the organizational structure. The ISCIII validated the proposal, distributed the funds to the selected nodes, and appointed Dr. Villena as general coordinator.

The structure of the project followed a similar pattern as the previous proposal and it can be summarized as follows, based on five strategic axes (instead of programs):

1. Coordination and governance
2. Samples and collections
3. R&D + i
4. ELSI and communication
5. Customer service and new markets

1. **Coordination and governance** (Coordinated by Cristina Villena, Majorca)
   (a) **General organization and strategy**. The network was organized around a directive committee assisted by an external advisory board. The coordination was based on a governance team with Dr. Villena as appointed coordinator and Jacobo Martinez (Valencia) and María Antonia Fortuño (Pamplona) as assistant coordinators.
   (b) **Monitoring and resources management**. Development and implementation of activity indicators were put in place in order to evaluate unit performance.
   (c) **Institutional relations** (national and international stakeholders).
   (d) **Teaching activities**. The main learning approaches were based on networking and thematic meetings. Yearly, the network used to organize a national congress and support a university master's degree in biobanking at the Catholic University in Valencia.
   (e) **Quality assurance management**. Through a commission, the network promoted the quality policy and common methodology and assisted their members to implement their policies according to international standards.
2. **Samples and Collections** (Coordinated by Andrés García, Salamanca)
   (a) **Catalog** (Samples and clinical data). Two main objectives supported this line of action: (1) to be able to identify and exploit the strategic collections of the network, which were the ones that were well-characterized, rich in

associated data, and stored in several centers (national distribution), and (2) to able to activate prospective collection circuits following a common set of quality standards.

(b) **Implementation of sample/information request management system**. Designed and developed in the former project, this was meant to be the interface where customers and biobanks met.

3. **Research and Development + innovation** (Coordinated by Roberto Bilbao, Vizcaya)

   The network identified three main areas for potential growth:

   (a) **Sample quality**. Search for new biomarkers that allowed to measure the quality (fit for purpose) of the samples stored and solved the questions posed by researchers about usability of the samples in new applications.
   (b) **New samples**. The technological advances were facilitating the study of conditions in ways never envisaged. New storage conditions, different sets of aliquots from a given raw sample, all that required quick adaptation, and biobanks need to be flexible and alert.
   (c) **Development and technological innovation**. The network as an innovation platform had the goal to be open to collaborate with different industries in the development of new technologies that could have an impact on the market and in operations.

4. **Ethical, Legal, and Social Issues** (Coordinated by Ana M Torres, Madrid)

   This program was of the utmost importance in the field. Biobanking activity is highly regulated, and modifications of the status quo have a direct impact on operations. On the other hand, interaction and alignment with our stakeholders in the legal, political, and ethical field are key to avoid and/or mitigate risks and stablish an ecosystem that potentiates biobanking activity.

   The main tools used by the network were:

   (a) Ethical and legal observatory
   (b) Communication and dissemination

5. **Customer service and new markets** (Coordinated by Jose Antonio López, Valencia)

The network as a service provider was oriented around their customers and their needs. The objectives of this program were: (1) getting to know our customers (actual and potential) and their needs, (2) evaluate how the network services solved the problems they faced, and (3) potentiate and diversify the market minimizing the competence.

In March 2020, the network initiated a special action to collect fully-annotated samples from COVID-19 patients. This special action included elaboration and distribution of specific guidelines on sample acquisition and management, ethics aspects to be considered, and specific training.

9.7 The New ISCIII Platform for Biobanks and Biomodels (2021–2023)

In August 2020, the Spanish National Institute of Health (ISCIII) announced a new competitive call for grants to "ISCIII platforms" to support R + D + I in Biomedicine and Health Sciences.

Its main objective is to support stable collaborative structures efficient and adaptable to research and innovation priorities, which would lead to a coordinated and immediate response to any scientific emergency that may affect Public Health.

Thus, this call is novel in several ways, firstly, it includes besides the biobanks, the concept of "biomodels" (in fact, it is renamed ISCIII Platform for Biobanks and Biomodels), encompassing, in addition to human samples (and their associated data), other models such as organoids, animal models of disease, and 3D biostructures. Furthermore, the new platform has as a priority the challenge of managing conventional human biological samples through virtual biobanks.

The new platform coordinator, Nuria Montserrat PhD from the Institute of Bioengineering of Catalonia (IBEC), has been appointed by resolution of the ISCIII Directorate. The coordinator is currently holding meetings to draw the future milestones of the platform as well as finalizing the Action Plan, The Steering Committee and General Indicators of Compliance.

9.8 Conclusion: The Most Important Lesson We have Learned

In this chapter, we have tried to introduce the main aspects of a long tradition of cooperative advances in biobanking from a nationwide perspective. As many other biobank network initiatives, we have had different external difficulties [27], committed mistakes, and achieved relevant successes, and during the journey, we have learned important lessons that can be summarized as follows:

1. Networking is an essential key to a better future in biobanking. Technical developments and the hope of more personalized medicine have renewed the need for high-quality tissue samples and derivates that are impossible to be obtained and managed by a single institution.
2. Biobank networks usually have a main initial promoter. However, to be sustainable, they should not be based solely on the irregular support of the main promoter, but also on maximum respect for the autonomy, idiosyncrasies, and freedom of each biobank.
3. In networking, attitudes (an open mentality for sharing) are more important than skills. Professionalization, clear contracts, and agreed upon procedures are extremely important and key elements, but networks exclusively based on contracts can ensure only short-term goals and usually depend on promoter support.

Networks also based on robust and friendly interpersonal relationships are a guarantee for long-term success.
4. A well-organized and operatively efficient nationwide biobank network is possible and should be a priority for every developed country.

References

1. Oosterhuis JW, Coebergh JW, van Veen EB (2003) Tumour banks: well-guarded treasures in the interest of patients. Nat Rev Cancer 3:73–77
2. Morente MM, Alonso S (2005) Current challenges of human tumour banking. Hematol Oncol 23:54–56
3. Meir K, Gaffney EF, Simeon-Dubach D et al (2011) The human face of biobank networks for translational research. Biopreserv Biobank 9(3):279–285
4. Watson PH, Barnes RO (2011) A proposed schema for classifying human research biobanks. Biopreserv Biobank 9(4):327–333
5. Gottwies H, Lauss G (2012) Biobank governance: heterogeneous modes of ordering and democratization. J Commun Genet 3:61–72
6. Hewitt R, Watson PH (2013) Defining biobank. Biopreserv Biobank 11(5):309–315
7. Morente MM, Fernández PL, de Álava E (2008) Biobanking: old activity or young discipline? Semin Diagn Pathol 25:317–322
8. Grizzle WE, Woodruff KH, Trainer TD (1996) The pathologist's role in the use of human tissues in research: legal, ethical, and other issues. Arch Pathol Lab Med 120:909–912
9. Cambon-Thomsen A, Ducournau P, Gourraud P-A et al (2003) Biobanks for genomics and genomics for biobanks. Comp Funct Genomics 4:628–634
10. Morente MM, Cereceda L, Luna-Crespo F et al (2011) Managing a biobank network. Biopreserv Biobank 9(2):187–190
11. Potocnik J (2005) New perspectives on the knowledge based bioeconomy: transforming life science knowledge into sustainable, eco-efficient and competitive products. Brussels: European Commission, DG Research; 2005. http://www.normalesup.org/~adanchin/lectures/kbbe_conferencereport.pdf. Accessed 31 Mar 2021
12. Tupasela A (2006) Locating tissue collections in tissue economies deriving value from biomedical research. New Genet Soc 25:33–49
13. Dhir R, Patel AA, Winters S et al (2008) A multidisciplinary approach to honest broker services for tissue banks and clinical data: a pragmatic and practical model. Cancer 113:1705–1715
14. International Society for Biological and Environmental Repositories—ISBER (2005) Best practices for repositories. I. Collection, storage, and retrieval of human biological materials for research. Cell Preserv Technol 3:5–48
15. Morente MM, Mager R, Alonso S et al (2006) TuBaFrost 2: standardizing tissue collection and quality control procedures for a European virtual frozen tissue bank network. Eur J Cancer 42:2684–2691
16. Morente MM, de Alava E, Fernández PL (2007) Tumour banking: the Spanish design. Pathobiology 74:245–250
17. Arias-Diaz J, Martín-Arribas MC, García del Pozo J et al (2013) Spanish regulatory approach for biobanking. Eur J Hum Genet 21(7):708–712
18. Nicolas P (2015) Spanish regulation of biobanks. J Law Med Ethics 43(4):801–815
19. Biobanking and Biomolecular Resources Research Infrastructure (BBMRI-ERIC). http://bbmri-eric.eu. Accessed 31 Mar 2021
20. OECD (ed) (2007) OECD best practice guidelines for biological resource centers: general best practice guidelines for all BRCs. OECD, Paris. http://www.oecd.org/dataoecd/7/13/38777417.pdf. Accessed 31 Mar 2021

21. Council of Europe (1997) Convention for the protection of human rights and dignity of the human being with regard to the application of biology and medicine: convention on human rights and biomedicine. https://www.coe.int/en/web/conventions/full-list/-/conventions/rms/090000168007cf98. Accessed 31 Mar 2021
22. Gonzalez-Sanchez MB, Lopez-Valeiras E, Morente MM et al (2013) Cost model for biobanks. Biopreserv Biobank 11(5):272–277
23. Lehmann S, Guadagni F, Moore H et al (2012) Standard preanalytical coding for biospecimens: review and implementation of the sample preanalytical code (SPREC). Biopreserv Biobank 10(4):366–374
24. Moore HM, Kelly AB, Jewell SD et al (2011) Biospecimen reporting for improved study quality (BRISQ). J Proteome Res 10(8):3429–3438
25. Riegman PHJ, Morente MM, Betsou F et al (2008) Biobanking for better healthcare. Mol Oncol 2:213–222
26. Red Nacional de Biobancos. http://redbiobancos.es. Accessed 31 Mar 2021
27. Devereux L, Watson PH, Mes-Masson AM et al (2019) A review of international biobanks and networks: success factors and key benchmarks—a 10-year retrospective review. Biopreserv Biobank 17(6):512–519

Chapter 10
Public–Private Partnership in Biobanking: The Model of the BBMRI-ERIC Expert Centre

Peter M. Abuja and Kurt Zatloukal

Abstract Biobanks for medical research provide access to human samples and associated data donated by donors or patients. They are typically established and operated by public institutions (e.g., universities, hospitals) and act as trusted partners for the resources, which are considered a common good for the advancement of biomedical research and healthcare. Although the ultimate expectation of donors and patients that their donation will contribute to improving healthcare can only be achieved if profit-oriented industry is able to access their samples and data, there are concerns whenever private companies generate profit based on public resources. In order to overcome this controversy, public–private partnerships, where joint efforts generate value both for the public and private sectors, could be an appealing solution. The BBMRI-ERIC-recognized Expert Centre (EC) is a model for such a partnership. ECs perform analysis of biological samples under highly standardized conditions and in accordance with ethical and legal requirements to generate high-quality data that can be used by industry for product development, and by the public, after a defined period of exclusive use for industry. Thus, expendable biological samples that otherwise could be used only by a small group of researchers are transformed into high-quality data that can be widely shared and used to advance biomedical research and development.

Keywords Biobanking for industry · Public–private partnership · Expert Centre · Trusted partner · Sample and data quality · FAIR data · Open data · Open innovation

P. M. Abuja · K. Zatloukal (✉)
Diagnostic and Research Center for Molecular Biomedicine, Institute of Pathology, Medical University of Graz, Graz, Austria
e-mail: peter.abuja@medunigraz.at; kurt.zatloukal@medunigraz.at

P. Hainaut et al. (eds.), *Biobanking of Human Biospecimens*,
https://doi.org/10.1007/978-3-030-55901-4_10

10.1 Biobanked Human Biological Samples and Associated Data as an Essential Resource for Industrial and Academic Research and for Improving Health Care

Advances in prevention, diagnosis, and therapy of human diseases ultimately rely on the availability of sufficient numbers of high-quality biological samples and data of patients. Biobanks are professional infrastructures for collection, preservation, storage, and providing access to human samples and associated data. They can be established, for example, in the context of specific cohort studies (e.g., large population cohorts) or within the health service [1–4]. Typically, donors or patients provide their samples and data to biobanks as donations, and biobanks are seen as a trusted, publicly funded environment that ensures the proper use of this precious resource for the benefit of certain patient groups or citizens in general. This expectation can only be met if biobanked samples and their associated medical data are efficiently used in high-quality research projects and their results lead to the development of novel products. This translation of a common good (i.e., donated biological samples and associated data) into commercial products, such as new diagnostics or medicines, requires smooth interaction of public and private sectors and transparent models for using public resources for private profit-making industry.

10.2 Major Hurdles for Industry to Work with Human Biological Samples and Data from Biobanks and Possible Solutions

10.2.1 Access to Samples and Data

Biotech and pharma industry need access to human biological samples and data to develop new products. For example, human biological samples are required for the identification of new diagnostic and therapeutic targets, preclinical research, defining disease indications and patient groups for clinical studies, and biomarker or companion diagnostics development [5, 6]. Therefore, providing access to biobanked samples and data is mandatory to meet patients' expectations that their donated samples ultimately contribute to improving healthcare. Nevertheless, the use of donated samples and data by industry to make a profit is viewed critically by the general public (and thus by potential donors) [7, 8]. It has turned out that one of the key factors for patients to donate their samples and data is implicit trust in public research institutions and clinics [9] and that this trust is significantly lower whenever donated samples and data are used in profit-oriented industrial research [10]. Apart from that, human biological samples are per se a costly and irrecoverable resource that should be used in the best possible way, avoiding conflicts of interest or interference with open competition.

10.2.2 Difficulties in Using Publicly Funded Resources for Profit-Oriented Research

Human biological samples and data are very often generated and preserved using public funds (e.g., research projects, healthcare systems, publicly funded biobanks). Releasing samples and data from the public domain for research that is essentially for-profit could therefore lead to a distortion of competition since the same sample cannot be given equally to all competitors that might profit from its use and from the public funding that contributed to its generation and preservation. Even a full cost compensation for accessing human biological samples and data cannot satisfactorily resolve this issue because the boundary between cost recovery (which is allowed in principle) for collecting, processing, storage, and releasing samples and data, and financial gain (which raises public concerns and is not allowed in some countries) cannot be clearly delineated. It is very difficult to correctly attribute the costs of the various processes involved in biobanking to a specific sample and dataset to be used in a project [11, 12]. Furthermore, the generation of biological samples and associated medical data in the context of healthcare involves many persons and institutions (e.g., surgeons, pathologists, oncologists, laboratory medicine personnel, radiologists, biobankers, etc.) who all have a stake in the biobanked samples and data. Therefore, their contribution should also be properly considered in cost recovery, which is not achievable in practice and constitutes, therefore, a potential source of conflicts that may delay or even block some projects. Moreover, the Oviedo Convention on Human Rights and Biomedicine [13] regulates a broad spectrum of issues in research that involves humans. In particular, Article 21 explicitly prohibits financial gain from using parts of the human body. Similar regulations exist in the USA (e.g., the "Common Rule" and the FDA Human Subjects Regulations [14]). On an international level, the UNESCO Universal Declaration on the Human Genome and Human Rights [15] stipulates these issues more generally. The OECD has issued guidelines that focus on the transparency and equality of terms of access to data generated from public funding [16, 17].

To overcome these problems of providing industry access to public biobanks, a model for a public–private partnership has been developed jointly by biobankers, patient advocacy groups, and industry representatives [18]. This model, called "Expert Centre" (EC), is designed to provide a trusted and quality-controlled environment that generates a win-win scenario for both the public and private sectors.

10.3 Public–Private Partnership (PPP) as a Model for Cooperation Between Healthcare, Academic Research, and Industry

10.3.1 What is a PPP?

The meaning of PPPs is somewhat vague since they span a wide range of quite diverse concepts ranging from simple bilateral collaborations to large projects dedicated to generating infrastructures (both physical and organizational) on the European or even global level [19].

In biomedical research and biobanking, PPPs may, for example, aim at developing joint expertise, knowledge, and resources thereby combining the specific assets of the public and the private partners, and so boosting the effectiveness of the innovation process. They come in many variations according to the need they should address [19], ranging from bilateral, small-scale cooperations to large multi-partner, e.g., national or Europe-wide, cooperations. The latter, like the Innovative Medicines Initiative [20], are specifically designed to advance research and development in the biomedical sciences throughout Europe, where the role of the public sector regarding trust and sustainability is emphasized [21].

10.3.2 How can a PPP Work for Biobanks and Industry?

Biobanks are typically established and operated by the public sector. There are however also privately owned and operated biobanks and some big pharma companies operate their own biobanks for their in-house research and development. In this chapter, we focus on public sector biobanks [18, 22].

PPPs in the context of biobanks can complement the large capacities and resources of the notoriously underfunded not-for-profit sector (academic research, public healthcare) with the financial resources of the for-profit-sector (industrial research and development) which would lead to a situation where both sides benefit, provided the legal and ethical issues can be solved. Such a PPP would contribute to sustainable funding of biobanks and provide access to samples/data and transfer of knowledge to private companies. PPPs can also avoid the stigma of selling samples to industry since they can remain in the not-for-profit environment and are transformed into data which are made accessible to the private partner. This enables the generation of data to build a growing public resource that conforms to the FAIR (findable, accessible, interoperable, reusable) principles [23, 24] and is of value both for the private and public partners. Hämäläinen and coworkers have performed a survey of the interaction of European biobanks with industry [22]. They found that most interactions are structured as research collaborations, which resemble PPPs at least to some extent.

10.4 The BBMRI-ERIC Expert Centre Model: A Solution for Many Issues in Biomedical Research

Already during the preparatory phase of the European research infrastructure for Biobanks and BioMolecular resources (BBMRI-ERIC) [25, 26], a PPP (the so-called EC) involving a trusted intermediate was proposed jointly by biobanks, the industry, and patient organizations [7, 18]. The EC performs the analyses of biobanked samples according to the state-of-the art, guarantees privacy and quality, considers pertinent legal and ethical necessities, and, in addition, the sustained public availability of the resulting data according to the FAIR principles [23, 24]. In this context, the EC transforms the biological samples of biobanks into high-quality data that can be jointly used by the private partner and the public.

The concept of the BBMRI-ERIC Expert Centre (EC) model involves:

1. *a not-for-profit public provider of human biological samples and data* that have been donated by patients with the implicit intention of supporting biomedical research. The public partner additionally provides medical knowledge and expertise (e.g., specific expertise of pathologists for selection and preparation of the most relevant tissue samples or clinical oncologists to extract relevant information from medical records) to the EC to optimize the analysis of samples and resulting data. Typically, this is a biobank associated with a healthcare provider and/or medical university or research centre.
2. *a private user of specific data and knowledge*. Typically, this is an industrial partner that pays for the costs of biobanking (not for the samples as such!) and analytical service. The private partner also contributes specific knowledge and expertise (e.g., specific quality requirements or industrial analysis platforms) to the project.
3. *an intermediate EC* that is trusted by both parties and performs the transformation of samples into data. The EC operates on a not-for-profit basis and guarantees to the provider of data and samples that privacy is properly protected and the samples and data are only used according to the informed consent and ethical clearance given. The pre-analytical and analytical workflows are performed according to the latest available standards and under supervision of the industrial partner. In this way, the industrial partner is in control of the quality of the data generated which is a prerequisite for further investments in product development based on these data. The data generated in the EC may be used by the private partner exclusively for a defined period, after which the data must be made available to the public domain.

Figure 10.1 shows the relationships between the key elements of the public and private sectors within an EC.

To make biobanks a resource that can legally, ethically, and technically serve industrial biomedical research and development as a partner, a BBMRI-ERIC-recognized EC must fulfill several requirements. BBMRI-ERIC has issued guidelines for the application to become an EC [BBMRI-ERIC-Associated Expert

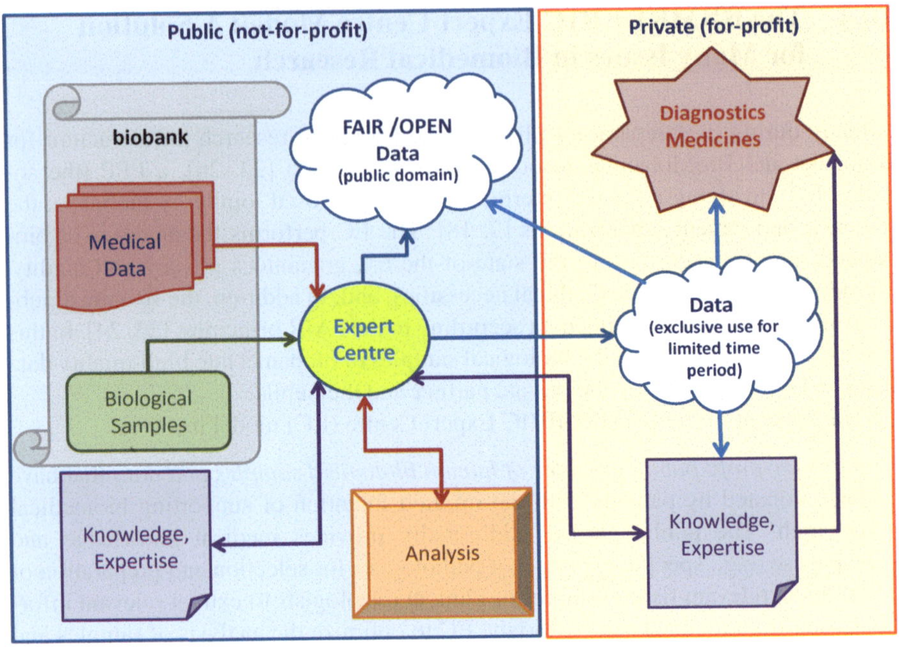

Fig. 10.1 The Expert Centre as a PPP of the public and private sectors

Centres/Trusted Partners, V3.0; www.bbmri-eric.eu] in which the key criteria for ECs are laid down:

1. It must be a trusted environment that guarantees patients' rights to privacy, and at the same time fulfills the donors' intention to contribute to the public good and advancement of medicine. This implies that patients' identities are not disclosed, neither directly nor indirectly. It thus combines the confidential medical and analysis data according to the research requirements and guarantees that this information cannot be used to (re-)identify the donors. Usually, this is done by coding and data aggregation, or by omitting parts of the data that are not required for research (principle of data minimization). The trusted environment, however, in principle retains all coded data, to allow reuse at a later time-point. In this context, special emphasis is placed on the prevention of reidentification of sample donors by combination of data sets from different research projects that use samples and data from the same donors.
2. It performs analyses on the samples in a highly standardized way according to the state-of-the-art thus delivering reliable data to the industrial partner in a transparent way. In this context, ECs pay specific attention to the requirements of a series of ISO standards for the preexamination phase, which are becoming increasingly important so that data generated meet regulatory requirements for future product certification (e.g., certification of in vitro diagnostics according to the European In Vitro Diagnostics and Medical Devices Regulation [27]). A

further requirement is that detailed information on analytical procedures, applied standards, and experimental conditions are made available to the partner since otherwise the data may not be used for product development or cannot be shared later with the public and reused according to FAIR principles. The latter point is actually the reason why the analytical laboratory should reside in the not-for-profit domain: industrial laboratories are certainly capable of performing analyses according to the highest standards however they often do not disclose sufficient meta-information on analysis, standards, and experimental conditions, which is a prerequisite for reuse of data in the public domain.

3. The main value generated by the EC is the transformation of biological samples into high-quality data that can be jointly used by the private and public partners thereby allowing a finite resource to be shared with a broad research community. The interests of the private partner are protected since for the financial contribution a period of exclusive use of the data generated is guaranteed to the private partner. After this period, data will be made available to the public partner to be further shared with the research community. There are several examples of PPPs that have successfully demonstrated how such models of limited data exclusivity work (e.g., Innovative Medicines Initiative).

As of May 2019, three Expert Centers have been appointed by BBMRI-ERIC (Fig. 10.2).

10.4.1 Advantages of the EC Concept

One advantage of this PPP model is that biobanks and ECs can be financially compensated for processing samples into data along the entire patient-to-data workflow and for the maintenance of their biobanking infrastructures without challenging ELSI principles or raising public concerns. The research community (both academic and industrial) can sustainably (re-)use the high-quality data for their own research thereby supporting the motivation of the donors to provide biobanks with human biological samples and data. Another benefit of the EC is that the public sector, in addition to the financial contribution, also benefits from the partnership by receiving expertise and knowledge from the industry partner. Conversely, the private-sector partner benefits from accessing medical and scientific expertise from the public partner (in a much more interactive manner than in typical consultancy relationships). Furthermore, knowledge and expertise, together with assured quality of the data, make the results of this research more reliable and valuable. Last but not least it should provide improved access for private users to public resources.

Sharing of anonymized data instead of samples is becoming a preferred practice, implying that the required analyses are performed according to the highest standards, and only analysis results (not original biological samples) and related metadata are distributed. Medical and analysis data can then be shared in a way that is tailored to the researcher's need while preserving the donors' privacy. This is

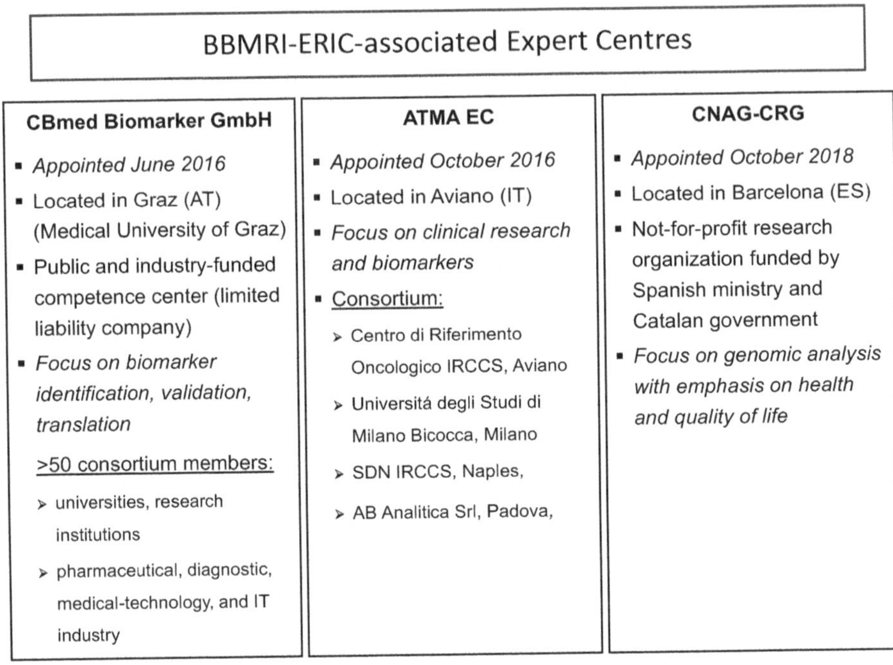

Fig. 10.2 Expert Centers recognized by BBMRI-ERIC (status May 2019)

particularly relevant since the transfer of samples outside the legal domain in which they have been collected may reduce the trust of the donors in the collecting biobank since, for example, using samples for other than the granted use (as specified in the informed consent and approved by research ethics committees) cannot be controlled effectively. Furthermore, most human biological samples contain the donor's genome which can be readily analyzed by next generation sequencing technologies revealing sensitive information such as risk factors of sample donors and their relatives and potentially allowing linking and reidentification of data. Another aspect is that there are several countries that have legal restrictions for sending biological samples to other countries for analysis. In this context, ECs could be a good solution for integrated sample analysis in international research collaboration since the need for sample shipment is avoided.

10.4.2 Sample and Data Quality

To ensure reliability and interoperability of analytical data, academic and industrial biomedical research requires access to high-quality human biological samples. The importance of sample and data quality is underlined by the "credibility crisis" in biomedical research that has disconcerted the scientific community [28, 29].

Furthermore, diagnostic errors contribute to 10% of patient deaths, and more than 50% of errors in laboratory tests can be attributed to pre-analytical factors, i.e., sample quality [30, 31]). Analytical performance gained further relevance in the context of personalized medicine, where most new drugs require a companion diagnostic test in order to select the right patients to treat [6]. In this context, the performance of a diagnostic test relates to the performance of very expensive drugs. These and other factors led to the series of ISO standards for the preexamination process and to new regulatory requirements such as the European Regulation (EU) 2017/746 on in vitro diagnostic medical devices [27].

Major efforts have been made in the last decade to introduce standards for sample quality, both for research and diagnostic applications, covering the whole pre-analytical workflow from sample collection to transport, processing, storage, retrieval, and isolation of various analytes (e.g., through the projects SPIDIA and SPIDIA4P [www.spidia.eu]). Previously, the importance of verification, standardization, and documentation of pre-analytical processes was insufficiently recognized, also because the focus was on optimization and standardization of the analytical technology itself. Meanwhile, standardization of the whole patient-to-data workflow has turned out to be of crucial importance and has a large impact on the data quality that industry (and also academia) requires. Therefore, ECs place much emphasis on sample and data quality, and processes have to meet the requirements of international standards. In order to demonstrate compliance with standards, proper quality management systems have to be in place. This may include certification or accreditation of ECs according to the relevant norms.

10.5 How Public–Private Partnership Models can Stimulate Innovation

10.5.1 Open Innovation, Biobanks, and Expert Centres

As PPPs, ECs implicitly foster collaborative research in the sense of Open Innovation by generating Open Data. This is due to the condition under which ECs operate, namely that the high-quality data they produce should be made available to the public domain following the FAIR principles, considering also the specific requirements of health-related FAIR data [23, 24]. In this context, it is important to emphasize that Open Data may not undermine ethical and legal requirements and specific access procedures for their use have to be applied. Since industrial partners support the sample-to-data conversion by paying for the sample analysis, they may also negotiate a period of exclusive use of the data generated within the EC. It is, however, desirable that this period is not too long. Similar provisions apply, of course, also for the academic exploitation of such data, e.g., for publications. Open Science benefits from EC-like PPPs since the publicly available data can serve further studies and minimize the need for reanalysis of original biological samples. This not only increases the use of the finite original biological samples but also avoids duplication of analysis efforts and finally speeds up the innovation process because research can build on existing data. At the same time, research based on Open Data is often more competitive since several groups may access the same data set and the intellectual property (IP) developed on the basis of Open Data has to be protected as soon as possible.

10.5.2 Management of Intellectual Property (IP)

Protection of IP is a prerequisite for the industry to invest in product development. Therefore, it is imperative for ECs to provide opportunities for the private partner to protect IP that emerges from data generated in the PPP. Protection of IP (which is not opposed to Open Data and Open Innovation [32, 33]) may require a grace period before data are made accessible to the public during which IP can be protected and, at least to some extent, a product developed and the market secured. Securing IP for an invention resulting from data generated in an EC that later becomes Open Data is not problematic since the openness relates to the data, not to the invention derived from them. However, subsequent controlled revealing of data and details (in the form of published patents, scientific publications, publicly available technical specifications) can lead to the generation of complementary assets (in the context of Open Innovation) as well as competing products.

There might also be situations in which EC-derived data per se do not lead to IP and therefore could be released immediately without compromising the innovative advantage of the private partner.

10.6 Conclusion

PPPs provide an environment for public biobanks that facilitates access to samples and data for industry and avoids concerns and legal barriers for using publicly funded resource for profit generation in private companies. BBMRI-ERIC-associated ECs are a specific type of PPP, which generate high-quality data as a common benefit for the public and private partners. In this context, it is critical that ELSI issues, particularly the protection of privacy of the sample donor/patient, are guaranteed and that biosamples and analytical technologies are of the highest quality. This is a prerequisite for the industry to use the data for further product development, and for the data to be widely reused (after a limited period of exclusive use for the private partner who has funded the analysis) by the scientific community. Insofar, ECs may become a prototype for FAIR and Open Data producers thereby stimulating Open Innovation.

Acknowledgments This work has received funding from the Horizon 2020 Research and Innovation Programme of the European Union, projects ADOPT BBMRI-ERIC (Grant Agreement No. 676550), CORBEL (Grant Agreement No. 654248), and the Austrian Federal Ministry of Education, Science and Research, project BBMRI.at [GZ 10.470/0016-II/3/2013]. We thank Dr. Penelope Kungl for critically reading the manuscript.

References

1. Riegman PH, Morente MM, Betsou F, de Blasio P, Geary P, Marble Arch International Working Group on Biobanking for Biomedical Research (2008) Biobanking for better healthcare. Mol Oncol 2(3):213–222
2. Asslaber M, Zatloukal K (2007) Biobanks: transnational, European and global networks. Brief Funct Genomic Proteomic 6(3):193–201
3. Hewitt RE (2011) Biobanking: the foundation of personalized medicine. Curr Opin Oncol 23(1):112–119
4. Simell BA, Törnwall OM, Hämäläinen I, Wichmann HE, Anton G, Brennan P et al (2019) Transnational access to large prospective cohorts in Europe: current trends and unmet needs. Nat Biotechnol 49:98–103
5. Hainaut P, Vaught J, Zatloukal K, Pasterk M (eds) (2017) Biobanking of human biospecimens: principles and practice. Springer International Publishing, Cham
6. Stumptner C, Sargsyan K, Kungl P, Zatloukal K (2019) Crucial role of high quality biosamples in biomarker development. In: Carini C, Fidock M, van Gool A (eds) Handbook of biomarkers and precision medicine. Chapman and Hall/CRC, Boca Raton
7. Biobanks need pharma. Nature 2009;461:448
8. Caulfield T, Borry P, Gottweis H (2014) Nature Rev Genet 15:220
9. Critchley CR, Nicol D, Otlowski MF, Stranger MJ (2012) Predicting intention to biobank: a national survey. Eur J Public Health 22(1):139–144
10. Clemence M, Gilby N, Shah J, Swiecikcka J, Warren D, Johnson J et al (2013) Wellcome Trust Monitor: Wave:2
11. Clément B, Yuille M, Zatloukal K, Wichmann H-E, Anton G, Parodi B et al (2014) Public biobanks: calculation and recovery of costs. Sci Transl Med 6(261):261fs45
12. Rao A, Vaught J, Tulskie B, Olson D, Odeh H, McLean J, Moore HM (2019) Critical financial challenges for biobanking: report of a National Cancer Institute study. Biopreserv Biobank 17(2):129–138
13. Convention for the Protection of Human Rights and Dignity of the Human Being with Regards to the Application of Biology and Medicine: Convention on Human Rights and Biomedicine; Council of Europe. Hum Reprod. 1997;12(9):2076-80
14. Bledsoe MJ, Grizzle WE (2013) Use of human specimens in research: the evolving United States regulatory, policy, and scientific landscape. Diagn Histopathol (Oxf) 19(9):322–330
15. UNESCO Universal Declaration on the Human Genome and Human Rights (1997) and International Declaration on Human Genetic Data (2003) UNESCO 2017
16. OECD (2007) Principles and guidelines for access to research data from public funding. OECD, Paris
17. Mascalzoni D, Dove ES, Rubinstein Y, Dawkins HJ, Kole A, McCormack P et al (2015) Eur J Hum Genet 23(6):721–728
18. van Ommen GJ, Törnwall O, Bréchot C, Dagher G, Galli J, Hveem K et al (2015) Eur J Hum Genet 23(7):893–900
19. Hodge GA, Creve C (2007) Public-private partnerships: an international performance review. Pub Admin Rev 2007:545–558

20. Goldman M (2012) The innovative medicines initiative: a European response the innovation challenge. Clin Pharm Ther 91(3):418–425
21. Goldman M (2012) Public-private partnerships need honest brokering. Nat Med 18:341
22. Hämäläinen I, Törnwall O, Simell B, Zatloukal K, Perola M, van Ommen GB (2019) Role of academic biobanks in public-private partnerships in the European biobanking and biomolecular resources research infrastructure community. Biopreserv Biobank 17(1):46–51
23. Wilkinson MD, Dumontier M, Aalbersberg IJ, Appleton G, Axton M, Baak A et al (2015) The FAIR guiding principles for scientific data management and stewardship. Sci Data 3:160018
24. Holub P, Kohlmayer F, Prasser F, Mayrhofer MT, Schlünder I, Martin GM et al (2018) Enhancing reuse of data and biological material in medical research: from FAIR to FAIR-health. Biopreserv Biobank 16(2):97–105
25. Yuille M, van Ommen GJ, Bréchot C, Cambon-Thomsen A, Dagher G, Landegren U et al (2008) Biobanking for Europe. Brief Bioinform 9(1):14–24
26. Vuorio E (2017) Networking biobanks throughout Europe: the development of BBMRI-ERIC. In: Hainaut P, Vaught J, Zatloukal K, Pasterk M (eds) Biobanking of human biospecimens: principles and practice. Springer International Publishing, Cham
27. Dagher G, Becker KF, Bonin S, Foy C, Gelmini S, Kubista M et al (2019) Pre-analytical processes in medical diagnostics: new regulatory requirements and standards. Nat Biotechnol 52:121–125. https://doi.org/10.1016/j.nbt.2019.05.002
28. Freedman LP, Cockburn IM, Simcoe TS (2015) The economics of reproducibility in preclinical research. PLoS Biol 13(6):e1002165
29. How science goes wrong (2013) The economist
30. Plebani M (2006) Errors in clinical laboratories or errors in laboratory medicine? Clin Chem Lab Med 44(6):750–759
31. Committee on Diagnostic Error in Health Care, Board on Health Care Services, Institute of Medicine, The National Academies of Sciences, Engineering, and Medicine (2015) Improving diagnosis in health care. Balogh EP, Miller BT, Ball JR, eds., National Academies Press (US)
32. Zacherl N, Zatloukal K (2017) Intellectual property issues in open science, pre-competitive research and open innovation. zenodo.org/record/580056/files/CORBEL-D8.1_Concept%20paper%20IP%20issues_May-2017.pdf?download=1. Accessed May 2019
33. Abuja PM, Zatloukal K (2018) Concept paper on new business models related to open innovation. //zenodo.org/record/1408808/files/CORBEL_D8.2_Concept%20paper%20Open%20Innovation_August-2018.pdf?download=1. Accessed May 2019

Chapter 11
The Future of Biobanking: Meeting Tomorrow's Challenges

Jim Vaught, Pierre Hainaut, Markus Pasterk, and Kurt Zatloukal

Abstract Biobanking has traditionally encompassed the collection, processing, and storage of biological samples and other specimens from environmental sources. Most of the procedures currently used by biobanks have involved processing tissue and blood samples. Formalin-fixation of tissue samples and storage at ambient temperature, and freezing blood fractions are the normal methodologies. However, recent developments in biospecimen management promise to revolutionize biobanking. Economic pressures have resulted in new storage technologies, including dry storage, which promise to reduce the high cost of freezer storage. New analysis platforms including genome-wide association studies and metabolomics have altered biospecimen processing schemes. Sample types have evolved to include circulating tumor cells and induced pluripotent stem cells. These developments will lead to the need for additional methods to assure their proper processing and storage for translational research studies. As these new developments evolve and international collaborations continue to grow, there will be an additional need to coordinate best practices and continue to perform biospecimen methods research to develop evidence-based practices. In addition to technical aspects, there are serious ethical and regulatory concerns that will require additional guidance, including consideration of issues around the return of research results to biospecimen donors, and reporting incidental clinical findings.

Keywords Biobanking · Biorepository · Biospecimen · Biospecimen research · Circulating tumor cells · Induced pluripotent stem cells

---

J. Vaught (✉)
International Prevention Research Institute, Kensington, MD, USA

P. Hainaut
International Prevention Research Institute, Lyon, France
e-mail: pierre.hainaut@i-pri.org

M. Pasterk
BBMRI-ERIC, Graz, Austria
e-mail: admin.dir@bbmri-eric.eu

K. Zatloukal
Medical University Graz, Graz, Austria
e-mail: kurt.zatloukal@medunigraz.at

P. Hainaut et al. (eds.), *Biobanking of Human Biospecimens*,
https://doi.org/10.1007/978-3-030-55901-4_11

11.1 Introduction

Various aspects of the future of biobanking have been highlighted and discussed in other chapters in this volume. In this chapter, we will bring together those concepts and discuss the major initiatives that we believe will comprise the future of biobanking and the challenges that will need to be overcome to realize the full potential of biobanking to support and transform the biomedical research infrastructure.

First, it needs to be reiterated that even the definition of biobanking is somewhat controversial [1], which complicates the discussion of its future directions and challenges. In addition, there are several types of biobanks including clinical or hospital-based and epidemiologic, as well as various types of basic and translational research biobanks. Biobanks can also hold collections of environmental samples. However, for the purposes of this volume, we have concentrated primarily on issues related to the major types of human biospecimen biobanks. The future of biobanking in this context will depend on consideration of several technological, ethical/regulatory, and other factors outlined in this chapter. Already, over the past 10 years, we have seen steady progress in the development of biobanks beyond the traditional model of freezing samples from pathology collections and research laboratories, with little consideration of the variables that can affect their stability and long-term utility. As the field develops more quickly in coming years, change will occur at a much faster pace. We are already, for example, seeing that the evolution of "-omics" including genomics, proteomics, metabolomics, transcriptomics are having significant effects on the technical, ethical/regulatory, and economics aspects of biobanking [2].

11.2 Future Technical Developments and Challenges

The evolution of biobanking as a recognized branch of scientific research [2, 3] has resulted in the recognition that, like other branches of science, biobanking requires an organized approach to developing and implementing technological developments. Traditionally two major approaches to biospecimen banking have been followed: formalin fixation and paraffin embedding (FFPE) in pathology laboratories; and freezing various liquid (blood, blood fractions, urine, saliva, etc.) and tissue samples for epidemiologic studies. Future technical developments will need to consider the aspects discussed below.

11.3 Biobanking Infrastructure

For many years the "infrastructure" of biobanks was mainly based on pathology collections of FFPE samples and frozen collections of tissue and liquid biospecimens. Although these biobanks could be large "freezer farms" or smaller collections within pathology departments or research laboratories, these models rarely varied from a technological viewpoint.

These traditional models are now changing and will continue to evolve. The most obvious of these trends is that the large freezer-based biobanks are recognizing that from scientific, logistical, and economic viewpoints, newer ways to process and store samples need to be developed. Two major advances are facilitating this trend: development of "dry storage" techniques that provide stable biospecimens of adequate quality for most analyses [4]; and alternatives to FFPE samples that are recognized by pathologists to be of similar or superior quality, such as PaxGene Tissue [5].

The future of such developments will depend on further biospecimen research to validate the long-term stability of samples processed and stored using these new processes. In addition, such advances will continue to evolve as different and smaller sample types are introduced into the biobanking realm, as discussed in the following sections.

11.3.1 Sample Types

Tissue, tissue microarrays, blood, urine, and saliva have been the typical specimens collected for clinical, basic, epidemiologic, and translational research studies. Newer specimen types include induced pluripotent stem (iPS) cells [6] and circulating tumor cells (CTCs) [7]. iPS cells, CTCs, and other single cell types are becoming significant tools for biomarker discovery and development as well as drug development and other biobanking-related applications. As these various new sample types are developed as research tools, biospecimen science principles will need to be applied as for all sample types, i.e., the optimization of collection, processing, and storage parameters. Pre-analytical variables will as for all specimen types be important to sort out.

In terms of sample types, see the review by Cole et al. [8] concerning trends in specimen use for cancer research. Overall there has been a trend toward the use of RNA-based samples and analytical techniques.

11.3.2 Sample Analyses

Genome-wide association studies, next-generation sequencing, and advances in proteomic analyses are among the analytical platforms that have revolutionized various research endeavors. What sample types and volumes/sizes will be necessary for newer analytical techniques, and what biospecimen research gap analyses and studies will be required as additional advances in analytic technologies occur?

11.4 Best Practices

As noted in Chap. 6, 2nd Edition a variety of biobanking best practices and guidelines have been developed over the past 10–15 years [9]. Although these documents have a number of common themes and agree in general on many of the technical and ethical/regulatory aspects of biospecimen collection and management, there are some significant differences. Most of these differences relate to national and international variations in the implementation of informed consent and other regulatory procedures. But overall there are two major problems with current biobanking best practices: the lack of research that results in evidence-based rather than empirical practices; and the lack of international cooperation and harmonization of practices.

Major organizations such as the International Society for Biological and Environmental Repositories (ISBER), the US National Cancer Institute (NCI), the European, Middle Eastern and African Society for Biopreservation and Biobanking (ESBB), the Organisation for Economic Cooperation and Development (OECD), the standardisation and improvement of pre-analytical procedures for in-vitro diagnostics project (SPIDIA), and the Biobanking and Biomolecular Research Infrastructure (BBMRI) have made significant contributions to the development and implementation of biobanking best practices [10, 11]. The early versions of these documents, particularly the technical aspects, were based on the experiences of early biobanking efforts and empirical evidence that particular practices led to longer term stability and quality of biospecimens. In terms of the ethical, legal, and social issues (ELSI), biobanking best practices have evolved from national and international standards and regulations that were develop based on the Helsinki and United Nations recommendations [12]. However, as biospecimen research has developed, it is now recognized that the future success of biobanking will depend on evidence-based practices [13]. This is a particularly important point since biomedical research, in general, is now and will continue to be more collaborative and international in nature. As more such collaborations evolve into biobanking networks it is important that consistent standards are developed to assure the consistent quality of biospecimens. In turn, consistent quality requires the consistent application of evidence-based best practices. And evidence-based practices will require more biospecimen research that is published in peer-reviewed journals, and constantly updated and reviewed to arrive at consensus opinions on the implementation of changes in biobanking practice. The US NCI Biospecimen Research Database [14] as well as ISBER's efforts in documenting biospecimen research publications, need to continue and expand to support the development and documentation of evidence-based practices [15]. This is not a trivial undertaking and will require the involvement of international organizations and biobanking experts.

A second aspect of the international cooperation and harmonization noted above is the need to better control the development and implementation of best practices, in order to provide new and developing biobanks and networks with consistent standards to follow. Currently, it is still the case that new biobanks and biobank networks tend to "reinvent the wheel" in at least some aspects of their planning and implementation. Often these missteps revolve around such critical issues as the design of information systems and informed consent processes that have not considered well-established approaches thus wasting valuable time and resources. The future development of successful biobanking efforts will depend on better international coordination of best practices. Organizations such as ISBER, ESBB, and BBMRI will need to take the lead in coordinating such efforts, especially as significant new biobanking efforts are being developed in, for example, China, India, and Africa [16].

11.5 Information Technology

Information technology (IT) advancements continue to provide new tools that assist in the necessary functions of tracking steps involved in collecting, processing, storing, and disseminating specimens, as well as linking analytical platforms with specimen data. Some of the issues that remain to be resolved are generally all in the area of agreeing on common best practices to allow the convenient exchange of data. "Big data" and the expanded use of electronic medical records will also become factors in the collection and analysis of biospecimen-related data.

Other issues that continue to be of concern and will need to be resolved in the next generation of biobanks:

- A consistent approach to developing common sets of minimal clinical data.
- Agreement on IT standards for biobanks, e.g., inventory, tracking, data collection and processing, electronic data collection.
- Better approaches to interoperability of IT systems and efficient exchange of data within biobanking networks and collaborations.
- Related IT issues in molecular epidemiology studies such as batch effects and statistical treatments with respect to various analytical platforms.

11.5.1 Web Resources

More international cooperation will be necessary to provide biobank and sample "locators," i.e., identify existing websites and promote international cooperation. As more studies involving biospecimens develop into networks and international collaborations, it has become more critical to identify methods to locate and obtain access to specimens and data, i.e., when allowable according to local and national rules and regulations and access requirements. Many such locators are available on the Internet, but a way to consolidate and provide access in a convenient way to international users is missing. ISBER created a working group specifically for this purpose [17] that will hopefully lead to improvement in the situation.

11.5.2 Sample Transport and Packaging

Over the past 15–20 years bar coding of samples has revolutionized biospecimen handling by speeding up all processes and reducing errors [18]. The transition from standard one-dimensional bar coding to two-dimensional symbologies such as Data Matrix was especially significant in that smaller codes and labels with more information could be used on the standard storage vials. Now additional advances are allowing RFID codes to gain widespread use in biobanks, with wireless tracking of samples and freezer function [19]. These efficiencies, when combined with advances in biobank automation (see Chap. 3, 2nd Edition), will provide for further cost savings and return on investment.

11.6 Ethical/Regulatory

Ethical, social, and legal issues (ELSI, see Chap. 7, 2nd Edition) are the most difficult to coordinate and standardize, i.e., when compared with the more straightforward and increasingly evidence-based technical biobanking issues. Below some of the issues that will be most challenging to resolve are outlined.

11.6.1 Return of Research Results and Reporting Incidental Findings

Patients and other biospecimen donors are increasingly asking for access to their clinical results. The role of biobanks and their associated laboratories in producing both clinical and research results means that the lines between the two are often blurred. Research investigators have been traditionally been reluctant to share their findings with specimen donors due to the preliminary nature of the results, and the uncertainty of the ultimate clinical utility of the findings. However, this scenario is likely to change in future biobank-supported studies.

Similarly, reporting incidental findings to biospecimen donors who may have not been diagnosed with such a disease, or had been seen for a different reason, is also becoming a point of discussion [20], due again to the blurred line between clinical and basic research studies. Samples may have been collected and examined by a pathologist for the initial diagnostic purposes, but then checked again by a separate pathologist for quality control for a research study. The question will be, as this discussion progresses, how to control the reporting of new incidental findings back to the original clinical team and patient.

11.6.2 International Collaboration

National and international biobanking networks and other international collaborations involving biospecimens have been discussed with respect to adoption of best practices and other standards in several parts of this volume. The scientific issues can be resolved with more consistent adoption of evidence-based practices. However, there are additional issues related to restrictions imposed in some countries concerning the export of biospecimens. It would be advantageous to international collaborations to establish more consistent access policies across international borders.

11.6.3 Informed Consent and Privacy

Many of the issues related to informed consent and privacy related to differences within and among countries concerning their application of local rules and regulations. Such rules and regulations are constantly changing and hinder international cooperation and coordination. In terms of more recent developments to accommodate the return of results, commercial use of samples, and privacy concerns due to new technologies, informed consent documents have been required to evolve to assure that specimen donors are fully informed of all eventualities concerning the use of their samples. In many instances, these concerns are also addressed in a more legal framework in material transfer agreements. However, again, the policies and procedures relative to these issues will continue to be challenging for international collaborations.

In terms of streamlining the consent process, CTRNet in conjunction with the University of British Columbia is developing a "permission to contact" protocol, in which potential biospecimen donors are informed about the potential for participating in research studies early in the process and asked for their permission to contact about such participation.

11.7 Other Issues

11.7.1 Economic Issues and Sustainability

See Chap. 3, 1st Edition for discussion of biobanking economics and sustainability. A future trend will be toward more formal business planning for biobanks, to meet ongoing funding challenges in research.

11.7.2 Biobank Networks

With the emergence in Europe, Asia, Australia, and more recently in Africa of major centers for biobanking networks and national coordination, can these trends be leveraged to promote more international cooperation and coordination? It is critical that as new biobanks are developed in emerging countries, they take advantage of the known best practices and avoid the pitfalls that tend to delay and reduce the efficiency and effectiveness of such efforts. See, for example, the review of challenges faced in the new H3Africa initiative [16].

11.7.3 Educating the Public

In countries where national networks rely on public funding and support, it is vital that biobanking initiatives be fully explained in terms that are understandable to the general public. Potential donors are generally supportive of biobanking when fully informed, but biobanking is not well understood by most of the public, so such informational initiatives need to become more prevalent. See [16, 21, 22] for a discussion of such efforts.

11.7.4 Publications

Publication of biobanking efforts such as the development of evidence-based practices has become more prevalent as biospecimen science has developed. However, the details concerning biospecimen management are typically not well-described in the peer-reviewed literature [23]. It is important that authors, editors, and publishers adopt standards for writing manuscripts with biospecimens as a major component. The Biospecimen Reporting for Improved Specimen Quality (BRISQ) and the REporting recommendations for tumor MARKer prognostic studies (REMARK) guidelines are examples of publication guidelines that are becoming widely adopted [24, 25]. BRISQ will need to become more widely adopted and modified over time in terms of the requirements for biospecimen handling details.

In general, it will continue to be important to promote the publication of biospecimen research articles to advance the field. Such articles tend to be published in a variety of journals including those devoted to clinical chemistry, epidemiology, and pathology. The NCI Biospecimen Research Database [14] is one important central resource for biospecimen research publications and includes search functions that allow the literature to be scanned for important biospecimen pre-analytical variables and other factors. Several meta-analyses have been published which summarize some of the major tendencies concerning such factors [13].

11.7.5 Education

Biobanking education and in general the "professionalization" of the field have gained momentum over the past decade. Several degree programs in biological resource management are in place, including at Catholic University Lyon and in other locales [26]. In addition, online tools are becoming available which allow biobanks to develop and manage their programs with advice developed by experts. Among these are ISBER's Biobank Assessment Tool [27] and the Biobank Resource Centre [28] web resource developed by the University of British Columbia and the (Canadian Tissue Repository Network (CTRNet) [29] allow biobanks to gather information to establish and operate a biobank. Such resources will be critical as biobanking continues to develop as a scientific endeavor.

11.8 Emerging Biobanking Markets and Technologies

In the April 2021 issue of *Biopreservation and Biobanking,* a new section was introduced: Emerging Markets and Technologies. As noted in the Editorial by Gupta and Brooks [30]:

> We are now in an era that was once thought of as science fiction. Although biobanks are often associated with research, the application and concepts stemming from this sector have fueled a new generation of technologies geared at providing direct-to-consumer solutions in emerging markets across the globe. Examples include services to help you better understand your wellness, personalized biome products, targeted marketing campaigns, new data security infrastructure, and much more. This section will highlight the emergence of new markets and technologies that are either adopting or disrupting the biobank framework as they imprint on society. The solutions presented here are anticipated to help drive innovation within the biobank community.

11.9 Summary and Conclusion

In this chapter, we have discussed the questions that will drive the future direction and challenges for biobanking. Throughout this volume, we have tried to identify trends that will influence these directions and challenges. For decades biobanking has been a more or less stable set of practices involving fixed or frozen tissues and blood-derived samples. However, the last decade has seen significant changes in biobanking practices and standards. Many of these changes have evolved from the increasing need for national and international collaboration in translational research studies involving biospecimens. The need for adherence to best practices, as well as the evolution of increasingly sensitive analytical techniques, have also contributed to the critical need to treat biobanking and biospecimen science as full partners in scientific endeavors. As biobanking continues to change in the twenty-first century it is even more critical to pay close attention to developing and publishing policies and procedures that will lead to a more complete compilation of evidence-based best practices. International organizations such as ISBER, BBMRI, ESBB, and others will be critical partners in this venture.

References

1. Hewitt R, Watson P (2013) Defining biobank. Biopreserv Biobank 11:309–315. https://doi.org/10.1089/bio.2013.0042
2. Vaught J (2012) Biospecimens and biorepositories: from afterthought to science. Cancer Epidemiol Biomarkers Prev 21:253–255
3. U.S. National Cancer Institute Biospecimen Research Network overview. https://biospecimens.cancer.gov/about/researchnetwork/default.asp. Accessed 16 Feb 2021
4. Crowe JH (2012) Stabilization of dry storage materials. From Cryo 2011 symposium. Biopreserv Biobank 10:375. https://doi.org/10.1089/bio.2012.1043
5. The GTEx Consortium (2013) The genotype-tissue expression project (GTEx). Nature Gen 45:580–585
6. Grskovic M, Javaherian A, Strulovici B et al (2011) Induced pluripotent stem cells—opportunities for disease modelling and drug discovery. Nat Rev Drug Discov 10:915–929
7. Bettegowda C, Sausen M, Leary RJ (2014) Detection of circulating tumor DNA in early- and late-stage human malignancies. Sci Transl Med 6:224–234
8. Cole A, Cheah S, Dee S (2012) Biospecimen use correlates with emerging techniques in cancer research: impact on planning future biobanks. Biopreserv Biobank 10:518–525
9. Vaught J, Caboux E, Hainaut P (2012) International efforts to develop biospecimen best practices. Cancer Epidemiol Biomarkers Prev 19:912–915
10. Vaught J, Kelly A, Hewitt R (2009) A review of international biobanks and networks: success factors and key benchmarks. Biopreserv Biobank. 7:143–150. https://doi.org/10.1089/bio.2010.0003
11. Vaught J, Lockhart NC (2012) The evolution of biobanking best practices. Clin Chim Acta 413:1569–1575
12. World Medical Association: Declaration of Helsinki—ethical principles for medical research involving human subjects. http://www.wma.net/en/30publications/10policies/b3/. Accessed 26 Mar 2014
13. Engel KB, Moore HM (2011) Effects of preanalytical variables on the detection of proteins by immunohistochemistry in formalin-fixed, paraffin-embedded tissue. Arch Pathol Lab Med 135:537–543
14. NCI Biospecimen research database (BRD). https://brd.nci.nih.gov/brd/. Accessed 16 Feb 2021
15. Moore H, Vaught J, Engel K (2014) NCI biospecimen evidence-eased practices: a novel approach to pre-analytical standardization. Biopreserv Biobank 12:148–150
16. Abayomi A, Christoffels A, Grewal R et al (2012) Challenges of biobanking in South Africa to facilitate indigenous research in an environment burdened with human immunodeficiency virus, tuberculosis, and emerging noncommunicable diseases. Biopreserv Biobank 11:347–354
17. International Society for Biological and Environmental Repositories (ISBER). http://www.isber.org/?page=IRL. Accessed 16 Feb 2021
18. U.S. National Cancer Institute Biorepositories and Biospecimen Research Branch. Best Practices for Biospecimen Resources (2016). http://www.biospecimens.cancer.gov/bestpractices. Accessed 21 Feb 2021
19. Bettendorf E, Malenfant C, Chabannon C (2005) RFID technology and electronic tags to identify cryopreserved materials. Cell Preserv Technol 2005:112–115

20. Park JY, Fortina P, Kricka LJ (2014) Genomic test validation for incidental findings. Clin Chem 60:292–293
21. Wanzhen G, Ma G, Tan Y et al (2014) Factors associated with willingness to participate in biospecimen research among Chinese Americans. Biopreserv Biobank 12:131–138
22. Starkbaum J, Gottweis H, Gottweis U (2014) Public perceptions of cohort studies and biobanks in Germany. Biopreserv Biobank 12:121–130
23. Cheah S, Dee S, Cole A et al (2012) An online tool for improving biospecimen quality reporting. Biopreserv Biobank 10:501–510
24. McShane LM, Altman DG, Sauerbrei W, et al.; for the Statistics Subcommittee of the NCI-EORTC Working Group on Cancer Diagnostics (2005) REporting recommendations for tumour MARKer prognostic studies (REMARK). Eur J Cancer 41:1690–1696
25. Moore HM, Kelly A, Jewell SD et al (2011) Biospecimen reporting for improved study quality (BRISQ). Biopreserv Biobank 9:57–70. https://doi.org/10.1089/bio.2010.0036
26. The CTRNet Biobank Resource Centre table of biobank educational resources. https://www.ctrnet.ca/en/resources/. Accessed 21 Feb 2021
27. ISBER Biobank Assessment Tool (BAT). https://www.isber.org/page/BAT Accessed 16 Feb 2021
28. The CTRNet Biobank Resource Center. https://www.ctrnet.ca/en/resources/. Accessed 15 Feb 2021
29. Canadian Tissue Repository Network (CTRNet). https://www.ctrnet.ca/. Accessed 15 Feb 2021
30. Gupta R, Brooks A (2021) Introduction to new section: emerging markets and technologies. Biopreserv Biobank 18:45. https://doi.org/10.1089/bio.2020.29068.rjg

Index

P. Hainaut et al. (eds.), *Biobanking of Human Biospecimens*,
https://doi.org/10.1007/978-3-030-55901-4

C

M

N

O

P

Q

R

S

T

The manufacturer's authorised representative in the EU is Springer Nature Customer Service Centre GmbH, Europaplatz 3, 69115 Heidelberg, Germany. If you have any concerns regarding our products, please contact ProductSafety@springernature.com

Printed and bound by CPI Group (UK) Ltd, Croydon, CR0 4YY
22/09/2026
02221062-0005